Managing Breathlessness in the Community

Other books from M&K include

Working with Children who need Long-term Respiratory Support
ISBN: 9781905539697

Understanding Chronic Kidney Disease: A guide for the non-specialist
ISBN: 9781905539741

The Palliative Approach: A resource for healthcare workers
ISBN: 9781905539673

Better Patient Feedback, Better Healthcare
ISBN: 9781905539246

The ECG Workbook 2/e
ISBN: 9781905539772

Practical Aspects of ECG Recording
ISBN: 9781905539307

Timely Discharge from Hospital
ISBN: 9781905539550

Mentorship in Healthcare
ISBN: 9781905539703

Managing Breathlessness in the Community

Edited by

Janelle Yorke and June Roberts

Managing Breathlessness in the Community

Dr Janelle Yorke
June Roberts

ISBN: 9781905539-63-5

First published 2013

British Library Cataloguing in Publication Data

A catalogue record for this book is available from the British Library

Notice

Clinical practice and medical knowledge constantly evolve. Standard safety precautions must be followed, but, as knowledge is broadened by research, changes in practice, treatment and drug therapy may become necessary or appropriate. Readers must check the most current product information provided by the manufacturer of each drug to be administered and verify the dosages and correct administration, as well as contraindications. It is the responsibility of the practitioner, utilising the experience and knowledge of the patient, to determine dosages and the best treatment for each individual patient. Any brands mentioned in this book are as examples only and are not endorsed by the publisher. Neither the publisher nor the authors assume any liability for any injury and/or damage to persons or property arising from this publication.

To contact M&K Publishing write to:
M&K Update Ltd · The Old Bakery · St. John's Street
Keswick · Cumbria CA12 5AS
Tel: 01768 773030 · Fax: 01768 781099
publishing@mkupdate.co.uk
www.mkupdate.co.uk

Designed and typeset by Mary Blood
Printed in England by H&H Reeds, Penrith

Contents

Figures

Tables

Editors

Janelle Yorke, PhD, MRes, PGCE, RGN, Senior Lecturer, School of Nursing, Midwifery and Social Work, University of Manchester

June Roberts, MSc, FETC, RGN, Consultant Nurse Salford Royal NHS Foundation Trust and Clinical Respiratory Pathway Lead North-West England

Contributors

Iain Armstrong MSc, RGN, Nurse Consultant Pulmonary Vascular Disease, Royal Hallamshire Hospital, Sheffield

Sara Booth MD, MRCP, Honorary Consultant in Palliative Care, Cambridge University Hospitals NHS Foundation Trust; Associate Lecturer University of Cambridge, Honorary Senior Lecturer, Department of Palliative Care and Policy, King's College London, Honorary Lecturer University of Edinburgh,

Julia Bott, BSc, Consultant Physiotherapist, Virgin Care, Chertsey, Surrey, UK; Clinical Respiratory Pathway Lead South East England

Julie Burkin, BSc (Hons) Occupational Therapy, MSc Clinical Research. Occupational Therapist and Lead Practitioner, Long Term Conditions Service, Palliative Care, Cambridge University Hospitals NHS Foundation Trust Addenbrooke's Hospital, Cambridge

Jessica Callaghan, BSc (Hons) Occupational Therapy, Specialist Respiratory Occupational Therapist, Virgin Care, Respiratory Care Team, Farnham Centre for Health, Farnham, Surrey

Annette Duck, MSc, RGN, Interstitial Lung Disease, Nurse Specialist, University Hospital of South Manchester

Amy Gadoud, MRCP, MB ChB, BSc (Hons), Clinical Fellow in Palliative Medicine, Hull York Medical School

Miriam J. Johnson MD, FRCP, MRCP, MRCGP, MB ChB (Hons), Professor in Palliative Medicine, Hull York Medical School, The University of Hull; Honorary Consultant to St Catherine's Hospice, Scarborough, North Yorkshire

Alison Newey, BSc (Hons), Diploma in Respiratory Disease Management, RGN, COPD Nurse Specialist, University Hospital of South Manchester

Patrick White MD, Clinical Senior Lecturer in General Practice and Primary Care, Department of Primary Care and Public Health Sciences, King's College London

Foreword

Dr Iain Small, General Practitioner and Chair of the Primary Care Respiratory Society UK

Managing breathlessness in primary care is an important and often difficult task. The traditional approach to understanding and treating patients has been to start with the disease and then describe the process of diagnosis, treatment and reassessment. However, in real life people don't arrive with a label. Their breathlessness may be physiological, pathological, or both; and they may be suffering from more than one condition, albeit with similar risk factors, causes and symptoms. This makes it a challenge to ensure that they gain the best possible results from our involvement in their care, and the satisfaction of having done so effectively brings with it a real sense of achievement.

Fundamental to all we do to help our breathless patients is to get the diagnosis right. Only then can we understand and effectively measure the impact of their symptoms on their lives, and direct our efforts (and theirs) to the interventions that we know are likely to have the greatest positive impact.

Sometimes we will influence life expectancy, sometimes symptom severity, functional status or time spent in hospital, but we can always have an effect on the patient's quality of life, particularly as they approach the end of their lives.

The management of breathlessness includes a broad range of interventions, from activity and fitness to pharmacological treatments, rehabilitation, oxygen therapy and patient-specific support. It is important that we ensure that the best and most effective form of treatment is available to every patient, according to their particular needs.

Having been given the rare and rewarding privilege of looking after people with this most distressing of symptoms, it is incumbent upon us to understand and apply the lessons of clinical research and practice to our patients. This book is an invaluable aid in our efforts to do so.

Preface

Breathlessness is a very common and complex symptom in cardiac and respiratory illness. It varies according to the patient's underlying condition and the stage that condition has reached. Breathlessness may be reversible in early-stage illness but may become intractable as the illness progresses. In other words, breathlessness is not abated despite maximal medical therapy to manage the underlying illness such as bronchodilators and steroids in chronic obstructive pulmonary disease (COPD) or diuretics in heart failure. This situation presents community practitioners with the challenge of helping a patient to manage their breathlessness beyond the best medical care of the underlying illness. The focus of this book is the management of intractable breathlessness in the patient's home setting.

We have focused on four conditions – COPD, heart failure, interstitial lung disease and pulmonary hypertension – in which breathlessness is a key and often distressing and debilitating symptom. Although there are specific disease management methods for each of these conditions, there are also common breathlessness management techniques that are relevant to all patients, regardless of their underlying condition. Subsequent chapters address both the specific and general techniques.

We hope this book will be useful to the many practitioners who see breathless patients in their day-to-day practice and have a desire to improve the experience and clinical care that these patients receive.

1

Introduction to breathlessness and community management

Janelle Yorke and Patrick White

The term 'breathlessness' is generally used to describe the subjective experience of breathing discomfort. As a subjective experience, it is also influenced by psychological and emotional processes. Breathlessness is common in community clinical practice, and it is a particularly debilitating and distressing symptom in patients with cardiac or respiratory conditions. Doctors, nurses and other healthcare professionals (HCP) working in the community often have to assess and manage breathlessness.

Breathlessness is the key presenting symptom of chronic obstructive pulmonary disease (COPD) and of chronic heart failure, which are both predominantly managed in primary care settings. These conditions, taken together, affect about 5% of the Western world population (Simpson *et al.* 2010, Lloyd-Jones 2010). Breathlessness is also a key symptom of many less common diseases such as pulmonary hypertension, interstitial lung disease (ILD), and a range of other respiratory, cardiac and neuromuscular conditions.

As a presenting symptom in primary care, breathlessness demands accurate diagnosis and treatment of the underlying cause. Improvement in the symptom often indicates improvement of the underlying disorder. To this extent, breathlessness is also one of the markers of disease control. In COPD, for example, breathlessness is one of the main reasons for the patient to consult a clinician. The severity of the disease is defined by the degree of lung function impairment but it is the degree of breathlessness that drives clinical management, from the patient's and the clinician's perspective. However, in long-term cardiac and respiratory illness there is often a poor match between the level of breathlessness reported by a patient and the result of lung function tests (such as spirometry). This implies that a person's perception of the severity of their breathlessness is influenced not only by the degree of disease but also by a complex interplay of emotions, previous experiences, and social and environmental circumstances.

For patients with a chronic cardiac or respiratory illness, breathlessness can be severely debilitating and is known to cause fatigue. Breathlessness also impacts negatively on a person's emotional well-being, having been described as 'frightening' and 'distressing' (Booth *et al.* 2003, Bailey 2004). As a consequence, breathlessness significantly affects patients' quality of life. Yet, despite its high prevalence and associated co-morbidity, relatively few proven effective treatment options are available.

Breathlessness can arise in healthy individuals in response to benign stimuli, such as exercise or strong emotions (De Peuter *et al.* 2004, von Leupoldt & Dahme 2007), although these short-lived, reversible sensations are usually qualitatively different from the sensations experienced by breathless patients. Breathlessness without identifiable pathology can also occur in psychiatric disorders and in people with a high level of negative affect, panic or anxiety. This book focuses on breathlessness as experienced by patients with cardiac or respiratory disease. Psychiatric illness as a sole cause of breathlessness is therefore not included. However, it is important to acknowledge that psychiatric illness (including panic disorder, anxiety and depression) may be features of chronic illness in some patients. Where this occurs, the link between psychiatric illness and breathlessness will be discussed in the context of the underlying cardio-pulmonary illness.

Defining breathlessness

The medical term for breathlessness is dyspnoea, and both terms are now used interchangeably. The word dyspnoea is derived from the Greek *dys* (meaning 'bad' or 'difficult') and *pnoia* (meaning 'breathing'). Dyspnoea has been defined in terms of difficult or laboured breathing that is observable by another person, and breathlessness as the subjective feeling of laboured breathing with and without dyspnoea (West & Popkess-Vawter 1994). However, breathlessness (not dyspnoea) is the term used by patients. For the purposes of this book, breathlessness will be used as a generic term for breathing discomfort and will be considered to have the same meaning as dyspnoea.

The American Thoracic Society (ATS) provides the most widely accepted contemporary definition and states that breathlessness is 'a subjective experience of breathing discomfort that consists of qualitatively distinct sensations that vary in intensity. The experience is derived from interaction among multiple physiologic, psychological, social, and environmental factors and may induce secondary physiological and behavioural responses' (ATS 2012). This definition acknowledges both the physiological mechanisms involved in breathlessness and the person's psychological and behavioural reaction to the sensation of breathlessness, and provides the conceptual foundation for this book.

Reflection point Reflection point Reflection point

Think of a patient you have previously cared for in the community. In the light of the ATS definition, what factors might have influenced that person's experience of breathlessness?

Acute and chronic breathlessness

Patients who experience breathlessness as the result of long-term cardiac or respiratory illness generally endure long-standing chronic breathlessness with acute episodes or periods of increased breathlessness severity. The change from a persistent level of breathlessness to an acute episode may be precipitated by exposure to infection, noxious inhalants and weather changes, as well as by emotional factors such as fatigue, anxiety and depression. Change may also occur in terms of an elevation in baseline breathlessness that accompanies slow progression of the underlying disease. This book is concerned with people who have a long-term cardio-pulmonary illness, in whom breathlessness is generally a persistent sensation that may gradually worsen and be compounded by episodes of acute breathlessness.

Conceptual framework for managing breathlessness in the community

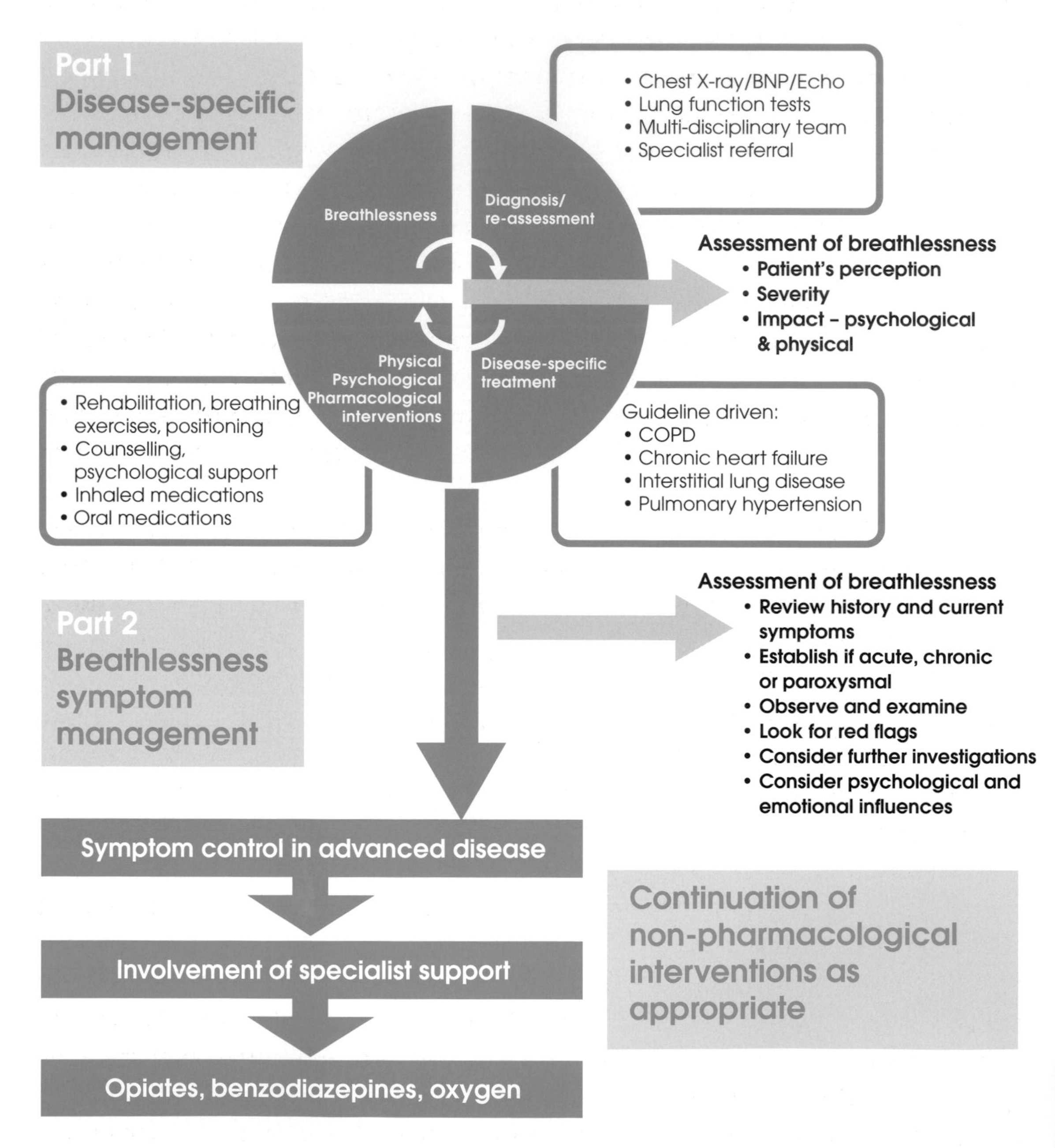

Figure 1.1:
Assessment and management of breathlessness in a community setting

The conceptual framework underlying this book reflects the multidimensional ATS proposed definition of breathlessness (ATS 2012). The framework therefore includes the physiological and psychological mechanisms involved in a person's perception of breathlessness. The framework starts with the presence of disease and its effects on the respiratory system (such as increased work, and stimulation of chemoreceptors and mechanoreceptors), leading to the sensation of breathlessness. The sensation is then perceived and interpreted by the patient. Perception is modulated by factors such as the patient's age, previous experiences and affect. The challenge posed by breathlessness, as it presents in a community setting, should be assessed in terms of the patient's respiratory rate, heart rate and hypoxia. In addition, assessing the underlying cause of the breathlessness will enable a practitioner to decide on the level of danger it represents and the urgency of intervention. From this point onwards, breathlessness may become a major reason for assessments, consultations and the provision of specific physical, psychological or pharmacological treatments (see Figure 1.1).

The above description aligns well with the 'total-breathlessness' model, which advocates a comprehensive, patient-centred approach to breathlessness assessment and management (Abernethy & Wheeler 2008). It applies the well-recognised total-pain model, originally articulated by Dame Cicely Saunders in the early 1960s (Ong 2005), to the field of breathlessness and addresses the patient's experiences of this symptom in the physical, psychological, social and spiritual domains. Total-breathlessness identifies the patient's experiences in the same four domains in an attempt to fully describe the suffering of an individual patient.

The total-breathlessness model begins with a physical assessment, including the cause of the individual patient's condition. The sensation of breathlessness can originate in the central and peripheral chemoreceptors, in response to an increase in carbon dioxide partial pressure ($PaCO_2$) and decrease in oxygen partial pressure (PaO_2) and pH (for more on this, see Chapter 2). The interpersonal domain of total-breathlessness considers the impact of the patient's condition on those around them and, in turn, the additional distress that these collateral effects produce in the patient. Spouses and other family members may all carry various emotional burdens, due to their relationship with the breathless patient, and patients themselves may feel the effects of damaged or strained relationships. Finally, with breathlessness, as with pain, patients may attribute many different meanings to the symptom, and the patient's religious or metaphysical beliefs may influence the extent of their suffering (Ong 2005).

The total-breathlessness model was originally designed to guide the palliation of breathlessness as a symptom. Here, we have expanded the model and applied it to the breathless patient not necessarily requiring palliation. Figure 1.1 (on page 4) incorporates the total-breathlessness model from a community care perspective and is underpinned by the concept of optimal disease management. The management of breathlessness in a community setting is schematically presented in two parts in Figure 1.1 – i) the disease-specific management cycle; and ii) breathlessness symptom management. The vast majority of breathless patients in the community are managed with disease-specific treatments. Before patients are considered for breathlessness symptom management, their disease-specific management should be optimal. Many of the physical and non-pharmacological interventions used in breathless patients should be prescribed as part of the disease-specific management cycle. Cardiac and pulmonary rehabilitation are very effective in moderate disease, significantly improving breathlessness, exercise capacity and quality of life (Lacasse *et al.* 2009). Some patients are extremely sensitive to breathlessness, which they find emotionally overwhelming and which can lead to crippling anxiety. Training in breathing management and anxiety control may be transformative in such patients.

The context of breathlessness in the community

Breathless patients make up a significant workload in the community or primary care setting but these patients mainly require disease management rather than symptom control. Approximately 30% of people who die of COPD in the UK are not seen by their GP or a specialist in the three months before their deaths (White *et al.* 2011). This suggests that many breathless patients who live in the community are likely to have sub-optimal control of their breathlessness.

In the UK, changes to the National Health Service (NHS) contract for General Practitioners (GPs), with the introduction of the Quality and Outcomes

Framework (QOF) in 2004, have led to the establishment of systems that can assist in identifying and managing breathless patients with advanced disease. These changes were further strengthened by the introduction of the Gold Standards Framework for the management of palliative care patients.

The QOF is a voluntary annual reward and incentive programme that has identified a set of target indicators in a range of domains. General practices score points according to their achievement against each indicator. This is relevant to the identification of severe breathlessness because the QOF encourages GPs to make registers of their patients with COPD and heart failure, and to record the Medical Research Council (MRC) dyspnoea score (Fletcher 1960) and spirometry of their COPD patients every 15 months.

If they are participants in the Gold Standards Framework, these practices will keep lists of patients with severe breathlessness who have moved into the terminal stages of their lives, and lists of patients with severe breathlessness whose disease management has been optimised but who may require palliative symptom management. Using these registers, GPs can easily identify patients who might be suffering from intractable breathlessness despite optimal treatment of their underlying disease. Such patients should be assessed to explore the potential for using symptom-alleviating interventions (such as non-pharmacological treatments and opiates) in an attempt to keep them comfortable whilst remaining in their own homes.

The National End of Life (EOL) Care Pathway (DH 2008) sets out a number of strategies to guide best practice for people nearing the end of life, of which being free of pain and other distressing symptoms (such as breathlessness) is key. The pathway aims to ensure that high-quality, person-centred care is provided, which is well planned, coordinated and monitored, while being responsive to the individual's needs and wishes.

More details on EOL care can be found in Chapter 10.

Reflection point

Consider how you might identify a person with cardio-respiratory disease who could be approaching the end of their life. What could you do to ensure that their care is optimised and co-ordinated?

Summary

The premise of this book is that breathlessness is a complex subjective experience that arises from multiple interactions between physiological, psychological, social and environmental factors (ATS 2012). Breathlessness is a prevalent symptom in many cardio-pulmonary conditions. Although each condition involves specific factors, many of the experiences described by patients and many management techniques are transferable between different diseases. A key factor in the assessment and management of breathlessness is to ensure that the patient's underlying disease is optimally managed. A number of pharmacological and non-pharmacological treatment options are available but the evidence base for many of these is limited.

References

Abernethy, A.P. & Wheeler, J.L. (2008). Total dyspnoea. *Current Opinion and Supportive Palliative Care.* **2** (2), 110–13.

American Thoracic Society (ATS). (2012). Update on the mechanisms, assessment, and management of Dyspnoea. *American Journal of Respiratory Critical Care Medicine.* **185**, 435–52.

Bailey, P.H. (2004). The Dyspnoea-anxiety-Dyspnoea cycle – COPD patients' stories of breathlessness: 'It's scary when you can't breathe'. *Qualitative Health Research.* **14** (6), 760–78.

Booth, S., Silvester, S. & Todd, C. (2003). Breathlessness in cancer and COPD: Using a qualitative approach to describe the experience of patients and carers. *Palliative and Supportive Care.* **1**, 337–44.

De Peuter, S., Van Diest, I., Lemaigre, V., Verleden, G. & Demedts, M. (2004). Dyspnoea: The role of psychological processes. *Clinical Psychology Review.* **24** (5), 557–81.

DH (2008) End of Life Care Strategy: Promoting high quality care for all adults at the end of life. http://www.dh.gov.uk/prod_consum_dh/groups/dh_digitalassets/@dh/@en/documents/digitalasset/dh_086345.pdf Accessed online 4/1/13.

Fletcher, C. (1960). Standardised questionnaire on respiratory symptoms: a statement prepared and approved by the MRC Committee on the aetiology of chronic bronchitis (MRC breathlessness score). *British Medical Journal.* **2**, 1665.

Lacasse, Y., Goldstein, R., Lasserson, T.J. & Martin, S. (2009). Pulmonary rehabilitation for chronic obstructive pulmonary disease. The Cochrane Library. DOI: 10.1002/14651858.CD003793.pub2.

Lloyd-Jones, D., Adams, R.J., Brown, T.M., Carnethon, M., Dai, S., De Simone, G., Ferguson, T.B., Ford, E., Furie, K., Gillespie, C., Go, A., Greenlund, K., Haase, N., Hailpern, S., Ho, P.M., Howard, V., Kissela, B., Kittner, S., Lackland, D., Lisabeth, L., Marelli, A., McDermott, M.M., Meigs, J., Mozaffarian, D., Mussolino, M., Nichol, G., Roger, V.L., Rosamond, W., Sacco, R., Sorlie, P., Stafford, R., Thom, T., Wasserthiel-Smoller, S., Wong, N.D., Wylie-Rosett, J. (2010). American Heart Association Statistics Committee and Stroke Statistics Subcommittee. *Circulation.* **121** (7), e46.

Ong, C-K, (2005). Embracing Cicely Saunders's concept of total pain. *British Medical Journal.* **10**, 576–7.

Simpson, C.R., Hippisley-Cox, J. & Sheikh, A. (2010). Trends in the epidemiology of chronic obstructive pulmonary disease in England: a national study of 51 804 patients. *British Journal of General Practice.* **60** (576), 277–84.

von Leupoldt., A. & Dahme, B. (2007). Psychological aspects in the perception of Dyspnoea in obstructive pulmonary diseases. *Respiratory Medicine.* **101** (3), 411–22.

von Leupoldt, A., Riedel, F. & Dahme, B. (2006). The impact of emotions on the perception of Dyspnoea in pediatric asthma. *Psychophysiology.* **43** (6), 641–4.

West, N. & Popkess-Vawter, S. (1994). The subjective and psychosocial nature of breathlessness. *Journal of Advanced Nursing.* **20** (4), 622–6.

White, P., White, S., Edmonds, P., Gysels, M., Moxham, J., Seed, P. & Shipman, C. (2011). Palliative care or end-of-life care in advanced chronic obstructive pulmonary disease: a prospective community survey. *British Journal of General Practice.* **61** (587), e362–70.

2

Mechanisms of breathlessness

Alison Newey, Janelle Yorke

Breathing is predominantly an involuntary neuromuscular effort controlled by the respiratory centre located in the brainstem. It is important to understand the mechanisms of normal breathing and breathlessness because a greater understanding of these mechanisms may lead to better assessment and treatment for breathlessness. The first part of this chapter reviews the physiological dynamics of breathing in health and in altered states, discussing the functions of breathing in relation to physiological processes and the preservation of homeostasis. The second part provides an overview of the mechanisms involved in the experience of breathlessness.

Part I
The physiological dynamics of breathing

Normal breathing and maintenance of homeostasis

In health, the lungs are compliant, distensible organs, and under resting conditions there is little awareness of breathing. The rate of respiration will fluctuate to accommodate the requirements of the body during periods of emotional stress, physical activity or sleep, for example. The primary function of the lungs is the regulation of gas exchange. In itself, this feature serves to maintain the pH of the body within narrow parameters (between 7.35 and 7.45), thus ensuring that cellular or internal respiration can take place. A revision of this process is simplified here to contextualise the properties of breathing:

Glucose + oxygen = carbon dioxide + water + energy

This formula demonstrates that basic cellular respiration is a chemical reaction. Oxygen is taken up by the cell to combine with glucose, resulting in the release of energy, whilst carbon dioxide and water are excreted as byproducts. The internal environment of the body needs to be favourable for this reaction to take place. Temperature, pH and oxygenation, for example, are therefore constantly being monitored and adjusted by the body to maintain an optimum environment. This regulation process is called homeostasis, and three physiological factors are required for the maintenance of homeostasis:

1 A receptor, which receives information and transmits to the control centre
2 A control centre, which processes the information received from the receptor
3 An effector, which responds to the signal from the control centre

For the control of breathing, these factors are represented by the following components (West 1995):

1 Chemoreceptors in the aorta, carotid arteries and medulla oblongata transmit information about the oxygen and carbon dioxide levels in the body to the respiratory centre.
2 The respiratory centre receives information about the oxygen and carbon dioxide levels in the blood and the cerebrospinal fluid.
3 The intercostal muscles and the diaphragm are controlled by the autonomic nervous system to influence the rate and depth of breathing.

The activity of breathing can be considered as a combination of physiological processes (Guyton 1983):

1 Movement of gases into and out of the lungs: This is achieved by the action of inspiration and expiration.
2 Gaseous exchange at the alveolar–capillary interface: The thin walls of the alveoli and capillaries, along with the minute space between these two structures, allow gases to pass into and out of the lungs by diffusion. Loss of this feature (as seen in respiratory disease where the alveolar walls are damaged, or pulmonary oedema where the space between the alveoli and capillaries contains fluid) will lead to impaired gas exchange.
3 Movement of gases around the body: The gaseous exchange allows for oxygen and carbon dioxide to be transported to and from the tissues of the body.

4 Control of ventilation: The rate of breathing is determined by the autonomic nervous system in response to the body's acid-base balance.

In cardiac and respiratory illness, one or more of these factors becomes dysfunctional. This leads to altered patterns of breathing as a regulating feature of homeostasis.

Dynamics of the respiratory system

The thoracic cavity

The lungs are situated in the thoracic cavity or thorax. This cavity is enclosed by the ribs, the vertebral column and the sternum, and is separated from the abdominal cavity by the diaphragm. The thorax contains the lungs, the middle and lower airways (tracheobronchial tree), the heart, the great arteries bringing blood from the heart out into general circulation, and the major veins into which the blood is collected for transport back to the heart.

The chest cavity is lined with a serous membrane called the parietal pleura. The membrane continues over the lung, where it is called the visceral pleura. Because the atmospheric pressure between the parietal pleura and the visceral pleura is less than that of the outer atmosphere, the two surfaces tend to touch. Friction between the two during the respiratory movements of the lung is eliminated by the lubricating actions of the serous fluid. The pleural cavity is the space, when it occurs, between the parietal and the visceral pleura. The penetration of air into the pleural cavity from outside (as from a penetrating wound of the chest) or from within, by rupture of dilated alveoli (air sacs of the lung) or of a cyst, will produce a pneumothorax. A pneumothorax turns this cavity into a positive pressure chamber and collapses the lung, which in turn will lead to decreased oxygenation of the venous blood. The collapse may also have a deleterious effect upon the heart and it requires immediate medical attention. When people have a pleural effusion, they have fluid build-up in this lining.

Lung expansion and contraction

The 12 pairs of ribs form a protective cage around the soft lung parenchyma. The intercostal muscles and costal cartilage allow for movement of the ribs during inspiration and expiration, whilst the dome-shaped diaphragm muscle contracts and relaxes accordingly. The movement of the ribs is described as a 'bucket-handle' motion. The ribs move upward and outward during inspiration, increasing the lateral chest diameter, whilst the diaphragm contracts downward (West 1995), increasing the vertical chest diameter. Furthermore, contraction of the scalenii muscles pulls the sternum upwards and forwards (pump-handle action), increasing the antero-posterior chest diameter. The combination of these actions increases the volume of the thoracic cage in all dimensions – an active process that requires energy to be expended.

This increase in the volume of the thoracic cage creates a pressure gradient between the thorax (where the air pressure has decreased) and the atmosphere (where the air pressure has not altered). To restore equilibrium, air is thus drawn into the respiratory passageways until the pressures are equalised. However, stretch receptors in the smooth muscle of the airways also respond to this action by limiting any further inspiration. In health, the lungs can recoil back to their resting state. Expiration at rest is a passive motion and no energy is expended by relaxing the respiratory muscles under these conditions. This feature is relevant to obstructive respiratory disease patterns, in which the natural recoil of the lungs is diminished over time and accessory muscles are recruited to support expiration.

Central neurological control of breathing

The main drive to breathe comes from neurons in the medulla oblongata at the base of the brain. The neurons receive signals from central chemoreceptors on the medulla, and from peripheral chemoreceptors located in the bifurcations of the aortic arteries and the aortic arch. These chemoreceptors are responsible for feedback to the medulla oblongata in the brain and are sensitive to the levels of hydrogen (H+) ions in the blood or cerebrospinal fluid. The respiratory centre responds quickly to the variations in the pH level sensed by the chemoreceptors, and instigates corrective action to maintain homeostasis (West 1995).

Hydrogen ion concentration in the blood is inversely proportional to the pH value. For example, the lower the pH value, the higher the amount of H+ ions in solution. A decrease in pH (<7.35) indicates a build-up of H+ ions in the body (an acidotic state), which could be of respiratory or metabolic derivation. Similarly, a raised pH value (>7.45) indicates a decrease in H+ ions (an alkalotic state). A full arterial blood gas reading would provide greater detail to help determine a diagnosis and the origin of the pH imbalance, though this is not always straightforward. As a primary compensatory mechanism, the body adjusts the rate of breathing in an attempt to normalise the acid-base balance. Thus in an acidotic state, for example, the rate and depth of respiration will increase as the body tries to eliminate excess carbon dioxide, which is acidic when dissolved in the blood (West 1995). Figure 2.1 demonstrates these relationships.

If this primary mechanism is not sufficiently effective and the condition persists, the body introduces a secondary compensatory mechanism to buffer the altered H+ levels (West 1995). For some individuals, this situation becomes chronic and the sensitivity of the chemoreceptors to raised carbon dioxide levels in the blood is diminished over time. In these patients, the stimulus to breathe is determined by lower levels of oxygen in the blood (hypoxic drive). The British Thoracic Society (2008) issued guidelines for the emergency use of oxygen to advise healthcare professionals of the clinical objectives when administering oxygen to patients, especially those who may have a history of hypoxic drive and carbon dioxide retention. More details on the practical implications of hypoxic drive and oxygen therapy can be found in Chapter 4.

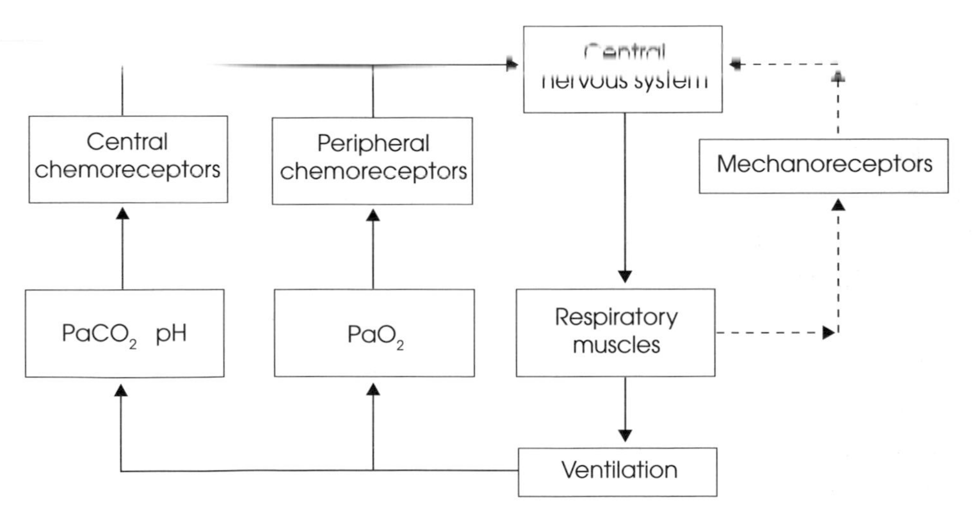

Figure 2.1: Schematic view of the central control of breathing

The left-hand cycle in Figure 2.1 shows that the central and peripheral chemoreceptors send information regarding the partial pressure of carbon dioxide of arterial blood ($PaCO_2$), and oxygen (PaO_2), and the concentration of hydrogen (pH), to the central neural systems. The respiratory muscles perform the motor commands sent by the central neural systems to achieve ventilation. In terms of system control, this component of breathing is a feedback controller, using information from chemoreceptors to increase or decrease the ventilation until the $PaCO_2$ and PaO_2 have returned to their respective set-point levels. The right-hand cycle illustrates the afferent discharge from respiratory mechanoreceptors that modulates the central command of respiratory muscles (West 1995).

Respiratory rate and I:E ratio

As discussed earlier in this chapter, the inspiratory phase of breathing requires energy to achieve contraction of the respiratory muscles. The normal respiratory rate for an adult during relaxed breathing is 12–18 breaths per minute, normally at a ratio of 1:1.5 or 1:2, inspiratory: expiratory (I:E) time. In an acute onset of breathlessness, the respiratory rate is increased and additional effort is required to maintain ventilation. This may be demonstrated by an alteration in the I:E ratio, with a longer expiratory phase as the work of exhalation increases. For some patients with a loss of elastic recoil of the lung fields, the expiratory phase may not be completed before it is time to take the next breath in, and this leads to small volumes of air becoming trapped in the lungs over time. Conversely, for patients with, for example, advanced interstitial lung fibrosis and loss of lung compliance, the I:E ratio may shorten, and inspiration (against the non-compliant fibrotic lung tissue) take as long as the recoil phase to give an I:E ratio of 1:1. Hyperventilation will also usually present with an I:E of 1:1. It is not routinely experienced as a result of illness but is more likely to be induced by fear or stress.

The rate and depth of breathing is determined by a multitude of short-term and long-term factors, as detailed below in Table 2.1.

Application of central breathing control to a person with COPD and 'hypoxic drive'

The central chemoreceptors are very sensitive to levels of carbon dioxide (CO_2) and they generally send signals to the brain that control breathing. The normal CO_2 level is 35–45mmHg or 4.7–6.0kPa. When CO_2 levels are high, a signal is

Table 2.1: Possible reasons for altered rate and depth of breathing

Chemical imbalance	Neurological issues	Changes in level of activity	Structural issues
Acid-base balance: Acidosis Alkalosis	Central nervous system (Respiratory centre, pulmonary stretch receptors and chemoreceptors)	Exercise	Thickened basement membrane: Oedema Bronchitis
Arterial blood gas tensions: Hypoxia Hypercapnia	Neurological deficit: Spectrum of motor neurone diseases	Pain	Alveolar loss of structure/traction: Emphysema
Acute illness: Septicaemia	Myasthenia gravis	Sleep	V-Q mismatch: Pulmonary embolism Atelectasis Pneumothorax Contusion, ARDS Inhaled foreign body
Ketoacidosis	Spinal cord compression	Impaired conscious level	Bronchoconstriction: Asthma Anaphylaxis
Anaemia	Guillain-Barré syndrome	Post-operative recovery	Chest wall restriction: Kyphosis Scoliosis
Clinical shock	Use of opiates		Pleural thickening: Malignancy Pulmonary fibrosis
	Anxiety Stress Fear		Loss of lung compliance: Pulmonary fibrosis Interstitial lung disease ARDS
			Loss of elastic recoil: Hyper-expanded lung fields

sent to the brain to increase the rate and depth of breathing in order to expel the excess CO_2. This mechanism means that CO_2 is our main drive to breathe. The peripheral chemoreceptors send a signal to breathe when the partial pressure of oxygen (PaO_2) in the arteries is less than 8kPa. The normal PaO_2 level is 75–100mmHg or 11.3–14.0kPa. This is known as the hypoxic drive. The hypoxic drive is much slower to respond to signals sent by central chemoreceptors so it only has a minor role in controlling breathing.

Some COPD patients have chronically elevated CO_2, perhaps greater than 100mmHg or 14kPa, and lowered oxygen level (PaO_2), less than 60mmHg or 8kPa. Many of these patients normally function with, for example, a PCO_2 of >7kPa and a PaO_2 of <8kPa. The hypoxic drive theory states that the high CO_2 makes the chemoreceptors tolerant of the high CO_2. For these individuals, CO_2 therefore ceases to be their drive to breathe. These patients are known as CO_2 retainers. In effect, this means that they are 'hypoxic drive' breathers. This is important, as giving oxygen to correct low levels can switch off the hypoxic drive and lead to worsening respiratory failure. This is known as oxygen sensitivity.

Arterial blood gases are not likely to be obtained in the primary care setting but a good understanding of normal values, and the implications of abnormal values, is essential for safe practice. Increasingly, however, community respiratory teams and home oxygen assessment and review services (HOS-AR) have portable blood gas analysers to enable them to take arterialised earlobe capillary blood gas samples. Non specialist primary care practitioners should not prescribe oxygen to people with COPD unless they have undergone blood gas analysis. Oxygen saturation levels using pulse oximetry are commonly used in the community and should be used to identify those with low saturations for referral. This is discussed in detail in Chapter 3.

Part 2
Physiological mechanisms associated with breathlessness

Breathlessness is largely attributable to the increased work of breathing during exertion (or at rest in severe disease) in order to eliminate increased amounts of CO_2. Respiratory sensations are appreciated at a conscious level. This means that information from receptors follows pathways so that it can be processed centrally and reach the cortex. A patient's perception of a symptom is therefore the end result of a series of processes, in which perception may not accurately reflect motor response.

Increased respiratory work and effort

The amount of work required to breathe depends on the individual's lung compliance and airway resistance. Lung compliance means the ability of the lungs to stretch in volume, relative to an applied change in pressure. The elasticity of the lungs (and hence their compliance) depends on the elasticity of lung tissue and the nature of the liquid lining the alveoli. When compliance decreases, the lungs are stiffer, and more effort is required to inflate the alveoli.

There is resistance to airflow during both inspiration and expiration. The energy required to overcome resistance represents the work of breathing. Under normal circumstances, breathing involves very little energy (accounting for 5% of metabolic rate at rest). Work or effort is required mainly to overcome airway resistance during inspiration. The effort involves muscular contraction in order to distend the elastic tissues of the chest wall and lungs and to move air through the respiratory passages. Part of the work of expanding the lungs and chest during inspiration is 'recovered': as the elastic structures recoil during expiration, air is passively expelled from the lungs.

Healthy people experience an increased sense of respiratory work during exercise. However, the sensation is usually rewarded by an increase in ventilation, even at high intensity, so it does not elicit an emotive response such as distress. In cardiac or respiratory illness, physiological adaptations that occur in health are disrupted and may lead to uncomfortable respiratory sensations. An increased sense of work or effort is present in several clinical conditions. Patients very commonly report that breathing 'takes a lot of effort', so this sensation is undoubtedly important in assessing clinical breathlessness.

Reflection point

How valuable is it to know the patient's baseline respiratory condition and how would this information form part of a respiratory assessment?

Fatigue and extremis

The respiratory muscles are able to meet the extra demand of the work of breathing up to the point of fatigue. This is largely due to the use of the accessory muscles in the neck and abdomen in an attempt to maintain inspiratory effort and thoracic expansion. A person utilising these accessory muscles typically sits or stands with arms leaning forward for support onto a chair, for example. This posture increases the thoracic space and helps them draw in more air. At this point, the person is becoming exhausted and blood gas tensions are likely to be affected by the lungs' failing capacity to take in oxygen and exhale waste carbon dioxide. Medical review is indicated if a person is too breathless to speak or cannot complete their spoken sentences.

Supportive treatment is delivered by means of controlled oxygen, bronchodilators, corticosteroids or diuretics in heart failure, and, in some cases, non-invasive ventilation (NIV) to restore acid-base balance and reduce the work of breathing. NIV for acute hypercapnic respiratory failure (ventilatory failure) is now commonly available in a secondary care setting, but is not yet available in community settings. It is important to have an anticipatory plan of care that includes the patient's wishes for, and the family's understanding of, end-of-life care. In this situation, non-pharmacological interventions (such as positioning, breathing control and energy conservation as well as palliation of symptoms) play a crucial role. Non-pharmacological and pharmacological management of breathlessness are discussed further in Chapters 8 and 9, and end-of-life care in Chapter 10. NIV is available now in the home setting for chronic ventilatory failure, primarily for those with either advanced COPD and chronic hypercapnia or progressive neuromuscular conditions, such as motor neurone disease or Duchenne Muscular Dystrophy, where the respiratory muscles are too weak to support breathing at night unaided and eventually during the daytime too.

An additional involuntary or voluntary method of assisting respiratory effort is the use of pursed-lip breathing on expiration. Breathing against a partially closed mouth helps maintain back-pressure within the airways; this mechanism serves to support airway patency for longer expiration to allow greater emptying; it may support the alveoli and optimise gaseous exchange. The individual will usually have adopted this positive end-expiratory pressure

(PEEP) without being aware of its physiological implications. In fact, PEEP maintains pressure in the airway so that the lungs empty less completely in expiration, thus increasing the amount of air left in the lungs following expiration. Such techniques are discussed further in Chapter 8.

Reflection point

Understanding intrinsic (auto) PEEP

Auto (intrinsic) PEEP involves an incomplete expiration before the initiation of the next breath and causes progressive air trapping (hyperinflation). This accumulation of air increases alveolar pressure at the end of expiration, which is referred to as auto-PEEP.

Auto-PEEP commonly develops in expiratory flow limitation (obstructed airway, such as in COPD) and expiratory resistance (narrow airway).

Once auto-PEEP is identified, steps should be taken to stop or reduce the pressure build-up. When auto-PEEP persists, despite management of its underlying cause, applied PEEP may be helpful if the patient has an expiratory flow limitation (obstruction).

Pursed-lip breathing is a method of applying PEEP; it does not cause auto-PEEP.

See Chapter 8 for further information about pursed-lip breathing.

Chest wall receptors and breathlessness

Afferent impulses from vagal receptors in the lungs (namely the pulmonary stretch receptors, irritant receptors and C-fibres) play a role in the sensation of breathlessness. Stretch receptors are stimulated as the lung expands and afferent information from the pulmonary vagal receptor is projected to the brain (O'Donnell *et al.* 2007). Receptors in the chest wall, in particular muscle spindles, primarily detect changes in the length of chest wall muscle and convey the information to the central nervous system.

Evidence for the role of chest wall receptors in modulating breathlessness has come from studies examining muscle vibration applied to inspiratory intercostal muscles during inspiration, and expiratory intercostal muscles during expiration. This mechanism has been found to decrease the breathlessness induced in both normal subjects and patients with chronic lung disease (Sibuya *et al.* 1994, Nakayama *et al.* 1998). It has been suggested that vibration of the chest wall activates muscle spindles and produces an illusion of chest wall movement.

Rapidly adapting, or irritant, receptors in the lungs are free nerve endings lying close to the surface of the airways' epithelium, at concentrated points where the airways divide (O'Donnell *et al.* 2007). These receptors can be powerfully stimulated by inhaling irritating gases and vapours, such as ammonia or cigarette smoke; and the receptors would obviously not encounter such physiological stimuli under normal conditions. Irritants (such as ammonia or smoke) or the receptors/nerve endings may be responsible for the changed patterns of breathing seen in asthma, culminating in the sensation of breathlessness and chest tightness.

C-fibres, located throughout the airways and lung parenchyma, respond to mechanical stimuli such as pulmonary congestion or emboli. Stimulation of C-fibres produces a pattern of rapid, shallow breathing and thereby plays a role in breathlessness sensation. C-fibre endings are attached to unmyelinated afferent fibres found close to the pulmonary capillaries, where they have been called juxtapulmonary capillary (type J) receptors (Eldridge & Chen 1995). The C-fibre endings or the type J receptors are stimulated by endogenously produced substances, which include histamine, some prostaglandins, bradykinin and serotonin. These substances may have a particular role in the breathlessness sensation associated with conditions such as pulmonary venous congestion with heart failure.

Hypoxia and breathlessness

Patients who are short of breath often state that they need more oxygen. Likewise, many healthcare providers' first instinct is to administer oxygen to the breathless patient. These actions reflect the widely held belief that breathlessness arises from lack of oxygen. However, it is a common clinical observation that hypoxaemic (or low blood oxygen) patients may not be breathless. Likewise, breathless patients may not be hypoxaemic, and correction of hypoxaemia may leave breathlessness unabated (American Thoracic Society 2012). The evidence for the role of hypoxia in the sensation of breathlessness is equivocal. From a clinical perspective, controlled oxygen therapy should be used to *correct hypoxaemia*, not breathlessness.

Oxygen administration in the community context is addressed in Chapter 3.

Hypercapnia and breathlessness

Research into the role of CO_2 in causing breathlessness has centred on the independent and combined effect of hypercapnia (or high blood carbon dioxide). Early studies suggested that breathlessness was a consequence of the effect of elevated CO_2 levels on respiratory muscle activity, as respiratory rate increases in an attempt to expel excess CO_2, and that stimulation of the chemoreceptor itself was not a direct cause of breathlessness. The seminal experiments conducted by Campbell *et al* (1969) on an experimentally paralysed subject and by Noble *et al.* (1970) on a patient with quadriplegia showed that large increases in end-tidal CO_2 produced no respiratory discomfort. For many years, it was therefore believed that the increased work of ventilation was the exclusive cause of hypercapnic dyspnoea.

More recent work has established that hypercapnia causes breathlessness independently of any associated reflex increase in respiratory muscle activity. Banzett *et al* demonstrated that ventilator-dependent patients with high-level quadriplegia, who lacked inspiratory muscle function, had breathlessness when end tidal CO_2 was raised above normal limits (Banzett *et al.* 1989). These investigators described the sensation of CO_2 induced breathlessness as 'air hunger' or 'uncomfortable urge to breathe'. The sensation of air hunger is likened to that experienced at the end of a prolonged breath-hold.

Respiratory failure

Although the underlying cause of illness may not be respiratory (see Table 2.1, p. 17), the illness may still affect the patient's breathing. Typically, in the early stages of an acute illness there is associated respiratory difficulty. Type I respiratory failure presents with a pH value within normal range, normal carbon dioxide level and an arterial oxygen level that has decreased to below normal value (<8kPa = hypoxaemia). The carbon dioxide level may even fall below normal to begin with when the patient is really struggling to maintain oxygenation, such as in uncorrected status asthmaticus. It is not unknown for an arterial blood gas taken at this point to dangerously confuse health care professionals, who may assume that a low CO_2 means the patient is improving.

If Type I respiratory failure progresses and remains unresolved, Type II respiratory failure will develop. At this stage, elevated levels of carbon dioxide (>6.1kPa = hypercapnia) and hypoxic levels of oxygen are demonstrated (Higgins & Guest 2008). These distinguishing clinical features indicate insufficient ventilation due to factors suggested in Table 2.1 (see p. 17). In a breathless patient, the clinical presentation of respiratory failure may represent acute changes in an already diagnosed long-term respiratory illness, where the body will deploy protective mechanisms in response to respiratory failure. Acutely, there will be an impact on the rate and depth of breathing (breathlessness).

If the situation persists, secondary mechanisms are introduced by the autonomic nervous system to maintain a normal pH and cellular respiration. The renal system regulates the secretion of bicarbonate as a secondary response to a change in the acid-base balance. Once these responses have become effective, the pH may be restored to within normal limits, whilst carbon dioxide and oxygen levels remain out of range. The body is thus said to have compensated for this imbalance.

The signs and symptoms of respiratory failure are non-specific and mainly reflect end organ dysfunction. Breathlessness itself does not define the presence of abnormal gas exchange. However, a high respiratory rate is one of the most sensitive signs of respiratory failure. For example, an increasing respiratory rate over baseline is more significant than an elevated but stable rate in a patient with COPD. Heart rate can rise due to cardiovascular distress but bradycardia in the context of falling oxygen saturations is an ominous sign.

Pulse oximetry reflects PaO_2 but tells us nothing about levels of $PaCO_2$ or pH. Rising $PaCO_2$ is usually a late or chronic manifestation of respiratory failure. The signs of CO_2 retention include headache, flushing, flap and tremor (Marieb 2001). In community settings, clinicians should remain alert to the new use of accessory breathing muscles. In particular, use of the inspiratory sternocleidomastoid muscles, and of the abdominal muscles on expiration, indicates excessive loading of the breathing muscles and strongly suggests a serious underlying respiratory problem. If not remedied, this may progress to respiratory muscle fatigue and failure and breathing exhaustion.

Reflection point

Consider how you would assess a patient for signs of respiratory failure in a community setting, when arterial blood gas analysis is not available.

Attention and breathlessness perception

Because breathlessness is a subjective experience, it can be highly dependent on emotional and cognitive processes. Psychological factors may alter the perception of breathlessness out of all proportion to the actual impairment in cardio-pulmonary function. This is not a new concept. Comroe (1966, p. 1) suggested that the experience of breathlessness involves 'the perception of a sensation and the reaction to the sensation'. Yet researchers have been relatively slow to investigate the psychological aspects of breathlessness.

It might be expected that individual differences in the perception of breathlessness would be partly related to differences in the attention paid to it by the breathless individual. A respiratory sensory gating system model has been proposed (Davenport 2007) and this was conceptually derived from the gate control theory of pain (Melzack & Wall 1965).

The sensory gating system model's first level is attentional modulation of gating. To perceive a respiratory sensation, the individual must first change their cognitive state and concentrate their attention on ventilation. Without this focusing of attention, the information about ventilation is 'gated' out of the cognitive centres. To make such a change in cognitive awareness possible, a significant change in information being relayed from the respiratory system is required.

The magnitude of attention threshold depends on a number of variables. These variables, or cues, may not be directly related to ventilation and may include affective states (von Leupoldt *et al.* 2006) and learning processes (De Peuter *et al.* 2004), which focus attention on or away from the sensation. The cortex and limbic system play a major role in the filtering process, particularly in the brain regions that process attention, thoughts and experience, and mediate emotional states, described below. If the signal strength from the respiratory system is stronger than the state dependent threshold, some of the information is processed in the somatosensory cortex – resulting in conscious awareness.

The second stage of respiratory perception involves affective awareness and evaluation (Davenport 2007). This entails deciding whether the breathing sensation has a comfortable or uncomfortable quality. This affective evaluation is crucial for voluntary, as well as involuntary, attempts to compensate for and control breathlessness.

Emotions and perception of breathlessness

As described above, afferent information received by the respiratory centre is filtered in the cortex. Emotional and cognitive processing is central to a person's perception of, and reaction to, breathlessness.

Studies involving neuro-imaging of healthy volunteers exposed to stimuli that induce shortness of breath have provided evidence of the involvement of the cerebellum (Evans *et al.* 2002, Banzett *et al.* 2000). In particular, the anterior insula is activated during episodes of induced respiratory distress. This is important because the insula is part of the limbic system, which is involved in aversive phenomena such as hunger, thirst, nausea and the perception of odours.

Taken together, neuro-imaging studies demonstrate a distributed network of limbic, paralimbic and subcortical brain regions associated with an increased subjective sense of breathlessness. This provides evidence of the role of emotional representation in breathlessness perception. Translating this evidence to the clinical scenario may reveal a more complex interplay of mechanisms. Teaching patients to better understand their breathlessness and what makes them anxious when breathless can reduce its impact on them. It's helpful to know that breathlessness has an effect on the brain, changing the way we think, feel and interpret experiences. Although the physical causes of breathlessness cannot be changed, we can therefore help patients to change the way they feel and take more control of their reaction to breathlessness.

Failure to recognise and address the emotional aspects of breathlessness may increase the patient's susceptibility to anxiety and depression, leading to increased symptoms, lowered physical function, poorer treatment adherence and reduced ability to self-manage (Yohannes *et al.* 2009). The relationship between emotions (such as anxiety) and breathlessness is discussed further in Chapter 3.

Summary

This chapter has reviewed patterns of breathing in health and as a result of acute or chronic illness, whilst also explaining the protective mechanisms that are employed autonomically to preserve homeostasis. Breathlessness is a subjective experience with underlying primary causes, and there is no single receptor or physiological mechanism that is responsible for the process of breathing. The evidence reviewed in this chapter suggests a relationship between respiratory work, chemoreceptors and mechanoreceptors, though the precise physical mechanisms of the sensation of breathlessness are still unclear. Alterations to chemical, mechanical or behavioural mechanisms can potentially lead to the sensation of breathlessness.

Brain-imaging techniques have been used to identify the brain structures involved in the perception of breathlessness. These images provide evidence for the activation of emotional and cognitive structures similar to those found in pain perception and other unpleasant experiences. Based on the available evidence, it is reasonable to assume that emotions play an important role in a person's perception of, and reaction to, breathlessness. This has important implications for assessment and management of the breathless patient.

References

American Thoracic Society. (2012). Update on the mechanisms, assessment, and management of Dyspnoea. *American Journal of Respiratory Critical Care Medicine*. **185**, 435–52.

Banzett, R.B., Lansing, R.W., Reid, M.B., Adams, L. & Brown, R. (1989). 'Air-hunger' arising from increased PCO_2 in mechanically ventilated quadriplegics. *Respiratory Physiology*. **76**, 53–68.

Banzett, R.B., Mulnier, H., Murphy, K., Rosen, D., Wises, R.J.S. & Adams, L. (2000). Breathlessness in humans activates insular cortex. *Neuroreport*. **11** (10), 2117–120.

British Thoracic Society (2008). Emergency oxygen use in adult patients. http://www.brit-thoracic.org.uk/Portals/0/Guidelines/Emergency%20oxygen%20guideline/THX-63-Suppl_6.pdf

Campbell, E.J., Godfrey, S., Clark, T.J., Freedman, S. & Norman, J. (1969). The effect of muscular paralysis induced by tubocurarine on the duration and sensation of breath-holding during hypercapnia. *Clinical Science*. **36** (2), 323–8.

Comroe, J.H. (1966). Summing up. In *Breathlessness*. J.B.L. Howell & E.J. Campbell (eds). London: Blackwell Scientific. 233–38.

Davenport, P.W. (2007). Chemical and mechanical loads: what have we learned. Pathophysiology of Dyspnoea in chronic obstructive pulmonary disease. A roundtable. *Proceedings of the American Thoracic Society*. **4**, 145–68.

De Peuter, S., Van Diest, I., Lemaigre, V., Verleden, G. & Demedts, M. (2004). Dyspnoea: The role of psychological processes. *Clinical Psychology Review*. **24** (5), 557–81.

Eldridge, F.L. & Chen, Z. (1995). Respiratory sensation. In L. Adams and A. Guz (eds). R*espiratory Sensation*. New York, USA: Marcel Dekker. 19–67.

Evans, K.C., Banzett, R.B., Adams, L., McKay, L., Frackowiak, R.S.J. & Corfield, D.R. (2002). BOLD fMRI identifies limbic, paralimbic, and cerebellar activation during air hunger. *Journal of Neurophysiology*. **88** (3), 1500–511.

Guyton, A.C. (1983). *Human Physiology and Mechanisms of Disease*. (3rd ed.) Tokyo, Japan: W.B. Saunders.

Higgins, D. & Guest, J. (2008) Acute respiratory failure 1: assessing patients. *Nursing Times*. **104** (36), 24–5.

Marieb, E.N. (2001). *Human Anatomy and Physiology*. (5th ed.) San Francisco, USA: Benjamin/Cummings Publishing Company Inc.

Melzack, R. & Wall, P.D. (1965). Pain mechanisms: a new theory. *Science*. **150**, 971–9.

Nakayama, H., Shibuya, M., Yamada, M., Suzuki, H., Arakawa, H. & Homma, I. (1998). In-phase chest wall vibration decreases Dyspnoea during arm elevation in chronic obstructive pulmonary disease patients. *Internal Medicine*. **37** (10), 831–5.

Noble, M.I.M., Eisele, J.H., Trenchard, D. & Guz, A. (1970). Effect of selective peripheral nerve block on respiratory sensations. In *Breathing: Hering-BreuerCentenary Symposium*. Porter, R. (ed). London: Wiley.

O'Donnell, D.E., Banzett, R.B., Carrieri-Kohlman, V., Casaburi, R., Davenport, P.W., Gandevia, S.C., Gelb, AF., Mahler, D.A. & Webb, K.A. (2007). Pathophysiology of Dyspnoea in chronic obstructive pulmonary disease: a roundtable. *Proceedings from the American Thoracic Society*. **4** (2), 145–68.

Sibuya, M., Yamada, M., Kanamaru, A., Tanaka, K., Suzuki, H., Noguchi, H., Altose, M.D. & Homma, I. (1994). Effect of chest wall vibration on Dyspnoea in patients with chronic respiratory disease. *American Journal of Respiratory Acute and Critical Care Medicine*. **149** (5), 1235–40.

von Leupoldt, A., Mertz, C., Kegat, S., Burmester, S. & Dahme, B. (2006). The impact of emotions on the sensory and affective dimension of perceived Dyspnoea. *Psychophysiology*. **43** (4), 382–6.

West, J.B. (1995). *Respiratory Physiology. The essentials*. (6th ed.) Philadelphia, USA: Lippincott Williams & Williams.

Yohannes, A.M., Willgoss, T.G., Baldwin, R.C. & Connolly, M.J. (2009). Depression and anxiety in chronic heart failure and chronic obstructive pulmonary disease: prevalence, relevance, clinical implications and management principles. *International Journal of Geriatric Psychiatry*. **25** (12), 1209.

3

Assessment of the breathless patient in the community

June Roberts and Janelle Yorke

Part I

Clinical assessment of breathlessness

Throughout this book, we can see that breathlessness is a common, distressing and disabling symptom that negatively affects emotional well-being and can completely overwhelm a patient's life. The multidimensional nature of breathlessness, and individual perceptions of its effects, mean that assessment has to include exploration of both physical and psychological impacts. However, the starting point remains accurate diagnosis of the underlying cause so that disease-specific management can be optimised alongside the physical and non-pharmacological interventions that can improve symptom control. This chapter introduces a systematic and comprehensive approach to assessing people presenting with cardio-respiratory breathlessness in community settings that underpins the assessment element of the adapted total-dyspnoea model (Abernethy & Wheeler 2008).

Initiating the assessment and gathering information

On initiating the consultation, it is important to clearly establish the presenting problem from both the medical and patient perspectives. Whether or not the patient has already been diagnosed with a cardio-respiratory condition, it is important to take a clear clinical history, as this will provide vital insight into the features of breathlessness that are most important to the individual, as well as information that may elucidate differential diagnoses. As breathlessness is such a subjective sensation, it is especially important to allow the patient to talk without interruption and to fully explain their problems in their own words. This can best be achieved by beginning the consultation with a general open question such as 'How are you feeling?'

It is vital to listen attentively to the patient's story and pick up on cues that warrant further attention – for example, how breathlessness impacts on their daily life, how it makes them feel, and any concerns and expectations they may have. Non-verbal cues (eye contact, facial expression, posture and movement) and vocal cues (rate, tone and volume) will provide further information on the patient's physical and emotional well-being.

Clinicians should sense-check their understanding of the situation with the patient and ensure that any concerns have been addressed before moving on to gather further information on the clinical history. Open and direct questions can then be used to establish medical perspectives (such as the chronology of their illness) and other diagnostically important features (such as the onset of breathlessness and any exacerbating factors). Additional background information should also be gathered to guide clinical thinking and govern next steps. This information should include:

- Past medical history
- Drug and allergy history
- Family history
- Personal and social history
- Systems review to include presence or absence of additional signs and symptoms.

Signs and symptoms

Patients with cardio-respiratory conditions endure persistent and progressive breathlessness compounded by acute exacerbations that worsen symptoms. The presentation of breathlessness can therefore be acute, chronic or paroxysmal (see Table 3.1). In addition, patients can be extremely sensitive to breathlessness, which they may find emotionally overwhelming. This can lead to crippling anxiety that further exacerbates breathlessness (see Figure 3.1). It is unsurprising then that levels of anxiety and depression are high in many cardiac and respiratory conditions. Co-morbid depression and anxiety are associated with increased mortality and utilisation of healthcare resources (Kim *et al.* 2000).

It can be difficult for patients and clinicians to differentiate between certain symptoms of anxiety and certain symptoms of cardio-respiratory disease (Maurer *et al.* 2008). However, it is important to include assessment for common signs of anxiety and depression because they are often unrecognised. If under-treated, they can lead to more symptoms, lower physical function, poorer treatment adherence and reduced ability to self-manage (Dowson *et al.* 2004, Maurer *et al.* 2008, Yohannes *et al.* 2009). Common signs of anxiety can be found in Table 3.2.

Table 3.1: Common presentations of acute, chronic and paroxysmal breathlessness in cardio-respiratory disease

Acute	Exacerbation of COPD, asthma or heart failure Atrial fibrillation and other cardiac arrhythmia Left ventricular failure Pulmonary embolism Pneumonia
Chronic	COPD Coronary heart failure (CHF) Interstitial lung disease (ILD) Lung cancer
Paroxysmal	Asthma, hyperventilation syndrome

Table 3.2: Common signs of anxiety

- Irritability and agitation
- Breathlessness or finding it hard to get a breath in
- Palpitations
- Dry mouth, butterflies in the stomach, feeling sick
- Light headedness and dizziness
- Tingling in the fingers and hands
- Tremor
- Sweating

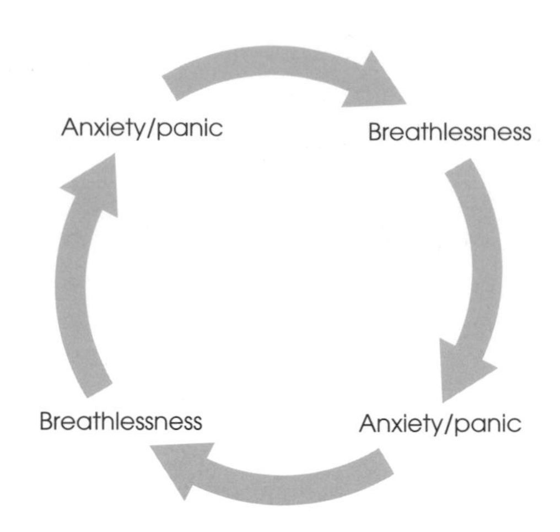

Figure 3.1: Breathlessness–anxiety–breathlessness cycle

The most common causes of cardio-respiratory breathlessness in the community (COPD, CHF and asthma) share many similar features. However, the presentation of the conditions, underlying precipitating factors and response to treatment differ (see Table 3.3). Red flag symptoms, such as haemoptysis in adult smokers, should also alert clinicians to the possibility of lung cancer, an important differential diagnosis in high-risk groups. Additional red flag symptoms for alternative diagnoses can be found in Table 3.4 (see page 34).

Table 3.3: Common features of asthma, COPD and heart failure

	Asthma	**COPD**	**Heart failure**
Age of onset	Usually under 35 years but can occur at any age	Usually over 35 years	Usually over 65 years
Smoking history	May or may not smoke	Usually current or ex-smoker	Often current or ex-smoker
Underlying risk/ precipitating factors	Genetic predisposition Occupational exposures	Smoking Occupational exposures Family history of emphysema – genetic predisposition (Alpha1 antitrypsin deficiency)	Hypertension Myocardial infarction History of heart murmurs Diabetes Mellitus Personal or family history of cardiomyopathy

Common symptoms and signs	Variable breathlessness, wheeze and cough Often worse at night and in response to clear trigger factors (often allergic)	Progressive breathlessness on exertion Morning cough with sputum Wheeze, especially during exacerbation Cyanosis, peripheral oedema, general fatigue and weakness in very severe disease	Progressive breathlessness on exertion Orthopnea and paroxysmal nocturnal dyspnea Cough with frothy sputum Weight gain and significant peripheral oedema General fatigue and weakness
Lung function	Variable Usually normal if well controlled Obstructive if uncontrolled or long-standing chronic disease	Obstructive, with little day-to-day variation despite treatment	Variably normal, obstructive or restrictive, depending on response to treatment
CXR findings	Usually normal but may be hyperinflated if exacerbation or poorly controlled	Hyperinflation	Enlarged heart Pleural effusions
Bronchodilator response	Good symptomatic and lung function response	Good symptomatic response Possible small improvements in lung function	No response
Corticosteroid response	Good lung function and symptomatic response	Limited lung function and symptom response when given as monotherapy May reduce exacerbation rate	No response

Increasing breathlessness in pre-existing conditions (such as COPD, CHF, ILD and pulmonary hypertension) could be due to general worsening of the underlying condition or an exacerbating factor such as a bacterial or viral infection or new cardiac event. Medication issues also need careful assessment, as non-adherence and inadequate inhaler technique are common and can result in poor control of symptoms and increased healthcare utilisation (Lavorini *et al.* 2008).

Table 3.4: Red flag findings in the breathless patient

Acute onset symptoms particularly associated with chest pain
• Confusion or agitation
• Significant weight loss
• Haemoptysis
• Tachycardia, bradycardia or arrhythmia
• Cyanosis
• Stridor
• Unilateral breath sounds

Reflection point Reflection point Reflection point

What features in the clinical history and physical examination would help you differentiate the specific cause of increasing breathlessness in a patient who had both COPD and CHF?

Carrying out a physical examination

Physical examination follows the clinical history and should proceed along the well-trodden path of inspection, palpation, percussion and auscultation. General observation and inspection of the patient can provide a wealth of initial information on current health status, particularly in relation to cardio-respiratory disease. These initial general observations can be done whilst talking to the patient and should be interpreted in the light of the clinical history:

- Does the patient look unwell?
- Are they breathless at rest?
- Are they unkempt? (Implying that breathlessness is affecting their daily activities)
- Are they in pain or distress?

- Are there signs of confusion?
- Are there signs of overt weight loss?
- Is the breathing rate/pattern normal?
- Is there excessive use of accessory muscles?
- Is there tracheal tug?
- Is there audible stridor/wheeze?
- Is central cyanosis present?
- Is peripheral oedema present?
- Are there signs of anaemia/pallor?

Vital signs

When assessing the breathless patient in community settings, three basic signs help the clinician assess the potential danger and urgency of the situation:

- Heart rate
- Respiratory rate
- Hypoxia.

Heart rate

The measurement of heart rate provides valuable data regarding the integrity of the cardiovascular system. The resting heart rate of a normal healthy adult should range between 60 and 100 beats per minute. Older adults with cardio-respiratory disease are particularly at risk of rapid, slow or irregular heart rate and rhythm.

The usual sites for measurement are the radial and apical pulses. The pulse should be carefully assessed for rate, rhythm, strength and quality. A 30-second count can be accurate for rapid rates, but if the pulse is irregular the count should be for 1 full minute. It is important to assess regularity and frequency of any dysrhythmia and determine the strength of the pulse: bounding, strong, weak or thready.

If measuring the apical pulse, use of anatomical landmarks will allow the correct placement of the stethoscope over the apex of the heart, where heart sounds will be heard most clearly. This can be achieved with the patient in a sitting or supine position by palpating the point of maximal impulse, which is located at the fifth intercostal space, to the left of the sternum, at the mid-clavicular line.

Auscultate for normal first and second heart sounds. A third heart sound may be found in heart failure but can be difficult to hear, even by experienced clinicians.

Respiratory rate – the neglected vital sign

Observation of respiratory rate and pattern is a simple, yet vital assessment, but it is also the least frequently and least accurately performed (Cretikos *et al.* 2008).

The normal resting respiratory rate of a healthy adult is 12–14 breaths per minute. A respiratory rate of above 20 is classed as tachypnoea and is therefore an abnormal result. Patients with long-standing cardio-respiratory disease may consistently be tachyopnoeic and only present with increased breathlessness either because of exacerbation or reduced exercise tolerance.

One of the easiest ways to record respiratory rate is to do it at the same time as taking the patient's pulse. Both pulse and respiration rate should be recorded for a period of at least 30 seconds. Counting the pulse rate for the first 30 seconds and the respiratory rate for the latter half of the minute means that both observations can be accurately recorded without the patient being aware that their respiratory pattern is being observed.

Respiratory pattern is rarely recorded, but the depth, regularity, symmetry and type of breath should be observed and considered in relation to the patient's history and symptoms. Shallow, rapid breathing may be due to bronchoconstriction, anxiety and/or a multitude of other causes. Rapid, deep sighing breaths may be in response to metabolic acidosis, such as ketoacidosis. Slow, shallow breathing may be due to opiate overdose or neurological dysfunction.

Hypoxia

Hypoxia is defined as a low level of oxygen in body tissues or organs, whereas hypoxaemia is low levels of oxygen in the blood. Cyanosis is the physical sign of hypoxia. The presence of central cyanosis is a far more significant clinical sign than peripheral cyanosis.

Peripheral cyanosis is the presence of blue extremities (such as fingers and toes) while the tongue remains pink. This is commonly seen in healthy people in cold weather, in Raynaud's syndrome and in the presence of peripheral vascular disease.

Central cyanosis is the presence of blue lips and tongue and represents arterial hypoxaemia. For central cyanosis to be present, the arterial PaO_2 must be less than 8kPa (SaO_2 of <85%).

Pulse oximetry is a relatively cheap, rapid and non-invasive method of monitoring the oxygenation of peripheral blood. Pulse oximeters measure the amount of infrared light absorbed by saturated and non-saturated haemoglobin. This gives an estimate of the percentage of saturated haemoglobin, which is an indicator of arterial oxygenation. In the community setting, pulse oximetry is a very valuable method of estimating arterial oxygenation and hypoxia. The infrared light shines onto a capillary bed adjacent to the skin's surface. The most common site is the nailbed of the fingers.

Pulse oximetry depends on a number of factors to ensure its accuracy, particularly adequate, pulsatile blood flow to the peripheries. It is important to note that the main limitation of pulse oximetry is that it does not measure carbon dioxide and so it should only be used to give an initial assessment of pulmonary ventilation. People with stable cardiac and respiratory illness who have persistent levels of oxygen saturation ≤92% may benefit from long-term oxygen therapy. However, they should be referred for formal assessment, including measurement of arterial blood gases, to confirm the presence of hypoxaemia and exclude carbon dioxide retention, which is a sign of Type II (hypercapnic) respiratory failure, also known as pump failure.

Importantly, there is also significant risk of harm if supplemental oxygen is given in acute situations to some people with cardiac or respiratory disease, particularly if it is administered at high flow. In these situations, oxygen (if required) should be titrated to maintain a target saturation of 88–92% (O'Driscoll *et al.* 2008). Once stable, the patient's need for oxygen should be re-assessed after about five to six weeks if the oxygen saturation remains ≤92% on two separate occasions (NICE 2010). For more information on the prescribing of oxygen, see the Home Oxygen Service Assessment and Review: Good Clinical Guide available at: www.pcc.nhs.uk and http://www.brit-thoracic.org.uk/Portals/0/Guidelines/Emergency%20oxygen%20guideline/THX-63-Suppl_6.pdf, and Chapter 4.

How pulse oximetry works and what it tells you

Following its diffusion across the alveolar capillary membrane, oxygen is carried within the blood by two methods: i) about 3% of the oxygen is dissolved in the plasma; ii) the remaining 97% is bound to haemoglobin in the red blood cells to form oxyhaemoglobin. Oxygen readily combines with haemoglobin and this reaction is fully reversible. Four molecules of oxygen can combine with one haemoglobin molecule.

Oxygen saturation is a measure of how much oxygen the blood is carrying as a percentage of the maximum it could carry (i.e. four molecules). If a haemoglobin molecule is carrying three molecules of oxygen, then it is carrying 75% of the maximum amount of oxygen it could carry. If a haemoglobin molecule is carrying four oxygen molecules, then it is 100% saturated.

Oxygen saturation is also referred to as SaO_2 and via a pulse oximeter as SpO_2. Acceptable normal range for SpO_2 is 97–100%. Patients with a known cardiac or respiratory condition may have a saturation level of less than 94% that is acceptable. It is therefore important that clinicians working in the community have access to medically recorded notes that state the acceptable pulse oximetry levels for individual patients.

Additional signs

Peripheral oedema is characteristic but not unique to HF and causes can be multifactorial. Patients with severe COPD and cor pulmonale also develop peripheral oedema. Oedema can vary in severity, from mild ankle oedema to severe pitting oedema of the legs and sacrum, which can be extremely uncomfortable and debilitating. Patients often have difficulty finding well-fitting, comfortable shoes, and the accompanying thin fragile skin is prone to injury and abrasion that heals slowly due to poor tissue perfusion. The resulting reduction in mobility and comfort can further negatively impact quality of life and compound psychosocial issues.

Finger clubbing is a poorly understood clinical sign and can be present in a number of respiratory conditions (see Table 3.5 below). It is important to establish whether this is a new phenomenon and how rapidly the alteration in nail shape has occurred. The answers to these questions may help determine the cause of the clubbing.

It is important to note that finger clubbing does not occur in COPD or HF. If present, it should therefore be considered as an indicator of co-morbid or alternative pathology.

Table 3.5: Cardio-respiratory causes of finger clubbing

Respiratory	Bronchial carcinoma Interstitial lung disease Bronchiectasis Lung abscess/empyema
Cardiac	Sub-acute bacterial endocarditis Congenital cyanotic heart disease

Further investigations may be needed to confirm or refute the findings of the clinical history and examination. These include:

- Chest X-ray
- ECG
- Echocardiogram
- B-type natriuretic peptide (BNP) and other blood tests
- Spirometry

Assessment of smoking history and relation to breathlessness

Smoking is the most important risk factor for the development of COPD, with around 50% of people who remain smokers in the longer term (to age 65 years and over) developing the disease over their lifetimes (Lundback *et al.* 2003). A smoking history of 20 pack years or more is significant. A pack year can be calculated using the formula:

$$\frac{\text{Number of cigarettes smoked per day x number of years smoked}}{20}$$

Around 40% of people with COPD are continued smokers, compared to just over 20% of people in the general population (Purdey *et al.* 2011). Continued smoking accelerates lung function decline, increases symptoms including breathlessness, and reduces the effectiveness of treatment. Stopping smoking is therefore a priority. The most effective intervention is intensive counselling with pharmacotherapy, which results in a one-year abstinence rate of 12.3% amongst COPD patients (Hoogendoorn *et al.* 2010).

Explanation and planning

Once the history and examination are complete, it is important to give the patient an opinion of what is suspected and a diagnosis if possible. A clear explanation for the suspected cause of breathlessness should be offered, along with discussion of the relative seriousness, expected outcome and predicted consequences. It is vital to elicit the patient's reaction to the diagnosis and explore any concerns before a mutually agreed plan of treatment can be negotiated. Where the underlying cause of breathlessness cannot be ascertained or diagnostic uncertainty remains, referral to a specialist for further assessment should be considered.

Summary

The multidimensional effects of breathlessness warrant a comprehensive assessment of any patient presenting with this problem in a community setting. The aim of the assessment is to uncover the underlying cause so that disease-specific management can be optimised, whilst introducing the physical and non-pharmacological interventions that can improve breathlessness symptom control as early as possible.

Part II

The usefulness of breathlessness questionnaires in the community

When implementing community-based interventions (both pharmacological and non-pharmacological) with individuals who are breathless, measuring breathlessness is an important part of assessment. A plethora of questionnaires for the measurement of patients' reports of breathlessness exist. Most of these questionnaires focus either on patients' accounts of their perceived breathlessness intensity or severity (direct measurement) or on how far the breathlessness limits their activities or their quality of life (indirect measurement). In order to thoroughly assess whether or not a patient's experience of breathlessness has changed in response to an intervention or due to a change in their underlying condition, the clinician needs to know what the questionnaire is attempting to measure.

A number of reviews have focused on measuring breathlessness in the clinical and research setting (ATS 2012, Bausewein *et al.* 2007, Dorman *et al.* 2007). Most breathlessness instruments have been developed and validated for COPD, and caution should be exercised when using questionnaires in populations other than those for which the instrument has been rigorously validated. The following section provides a critique of approaches to measuring breathlessness, and discusses the relevance of the measurement method to assessing and managing the breathless person in the community, as well as offering some example of commonly used measures. It should be borne in mind that this review is not exhaustive and covers only some of the possible tools available.

Measures of breathlessness intensity/severity

Single-item measures of breathlessness

The Numerical Rating Scale (NRS), Visual Analogue Scale (VAS) (Gift 1989, Mahler & Jones 1997) and the Borg Scale (Borg 1982) are the most commonly used instruments to quantify a person's perceived breathlessness severity/intensity. These scales are one-dimensional, single-question scales that are self-administered and quick to complete. However, there are a number of common problems with these scales, involving a lack of consistency with their use and methods of application. The issues to be considered include:

- What aspect of breathlessness is being measured
- The recall period being used
- The scaling range (e.g. 0–10 or 0–100)
- The use of different verbal anchors at each extreme end of the scale.

Because there are no standard principles to ensure consistent use and the scales have been adapted to measure different aspects of breathlessness (for example, 'bother caused by breathlessness', 'distress due to breathlessness' and 'uncomfortable breathing'), it is essential that the practitioner has a good understanding of the precise aspect of breathlessness that needs to be measured and how to apply the appropriate wording in a consistent way. These scales have also been used simply to measure 'breathlessness intensity' (for example, 'worst breathlessness' or 'average breathlessness', over a given time period, and 'breathlessness right now'). This inconsistency makes it difficult to critique single-item scales across different studies. However, it is essential that the wording used should be consistent for each individual patient for each assessment point. This will ensure that the same breathlessness concept is being measured over time.

The following section describes the three commonly used single-item scales VAS, NRS and modified-Borg.

Visual Analogue Scale

The VAS has been shown to be a valid instrument for assessing breathlessness for individual patients with cardio-pulmonary disease (Gift 1989) with good intra-rater reliability. Although easy to use, the two VAS anchors are unique to each individual, making comparisons between people difficult. In the community setting, where an individual's response to treatment or trajectory of breathlessness experience over time is the factor being measured, the ability to compare between patients is not a key factor. The VAS consists of a line, usually 100mm in length, with descriptors (such as 'not breathless at all' and 'extremely breathless') at opposite ends of the line. The breathlessness score is found by measuring the distance from one side of the scale to the level indicated by the patient. This method can make the assessment process more laborious and cumbersome than the NRS or Borg Scale, since the latter provide an immediate numerical response.

To use a VAS 100mm:

- Ask the patient to mark their perceived degree of breathlessness on the line
- Then measure from the right-hand end of the line to the patient's mark

The VAS has been shown to be equally valid when the scale is orientated from the traditional horizontal to vertical (Gift 1989).

Not breathless at all ——————▶—————— Extremely breathless

Numerical Rating Scale

The NRS consists of a line with verbal anchors at each extreme, similar to the VAS, but it also provides equally spaced numeric indicators (see page 43).

Example of a NRS 0 to 10:

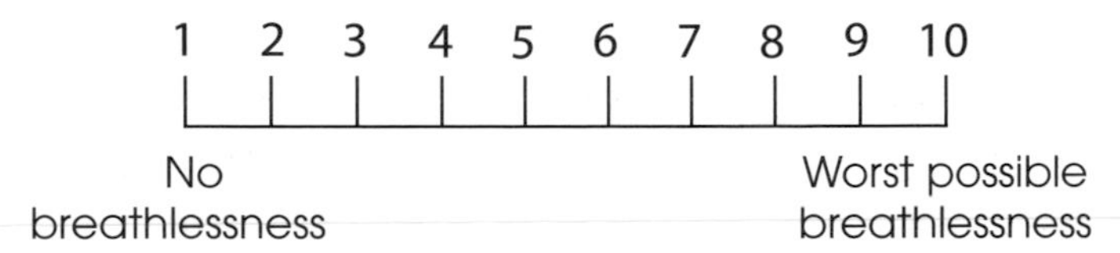

In research, the NRS has been used as an outcome measure for breathlessness less frequently than the VAS. However, it has been reported that in pain assessment the NRS is far easier for patients to use than the VAS (Caraceni 2001). It also requires less input from the assessor to obtain a score – once the patient has indicated a number on the scale, a breathlessness score is immediately available. Although correlations between the two scales are high, the NRS is more repeatable for breathlessness measurement than the VAS (Wilcock *et al.* 1999).

The Modified-Borg Scale

The Modified-Borg Scale is a 0 to 10 scale with verbal descriptors adjacent to specific numbers (Borg 1982). It was originally designed to measure the concept of perceived exertion during physical exercise, with ratings linked to heart rate ranging from 6 to 20. The scale was subsequently modified to include a 0 to 10-point scale to measure breathlessness intensity (Burdon *et al.* 1982) and is now the most commonly used form of breathlessness measurement, since it is both sensitive and reproducible enough to pick up short-term change, for example before and after an exercise test, with good intra-rater reliability.

To use the Modified-Borg Scale, say to the patient:

> Using the scale below, please indicate the severity of breathlessness you are currently experiencing.

0	**NOTHING AT ALL**	**5**	**SEVERE**
0.5	**VERY, VERY SLIGHT (just noticeable)**	**6**	
1	**VERY SLIGHT**	**7**	**VERY SEVERE**
2	**SLIGHT**	**8**	
3	**MODERATE**	**9**	**VERY, VERY SEVERE (almost maximal)**
4	**SOMEWHAT SEVERE**	**10**	**MAXIMAL**

Multiple-item measures of breathlessness

Dyspnoea-12

The Dyspnoea-12 (D-12) was designed to provide an overall score for breathlessness severity that captures the sensory quality ('physical' component) and the emotional consequences ('affective' component) of breathlessness (Yorke et al. 2010a). The D-12 quantifies breathlessness using 12 descriptors – 7 items deal with the physical aspect (such as 'My breathing requires more work' and 'I cannot get enough air') and 5 items focus on the affective aspect (such as 'My breathing is distressing' and 'My breathing makes me feel depressed').

A particular strength of this instrument is that it was developed using a large cohort of patients with COPD, ILD and CHF. It has subsequently been shown to possess validity and reliability for the measurement of breathlessness for COPD, asthma (Yorke *et al.* 2010a) and ILD (Swigris *et al.* 2010, Yorke *et al.* 2010b). The D-12 is quick and easy to use and provides a total score for breathlessness magnitude, using a simple summation of each item's score. Each item ranges from 0 ('none') to 3 ('severe') and there is a total scoring range from 0 to 36, with higher scores indicating more severe breathlessness. The reference period refers to breathlessness severity 'these days' to provide an index of a person's current experience. Although designed to provide an overall score of breathlessness severity, separate scores for the physical and affective components can also be calculated.

Indirect/Impact measures of breathlessness

Breathless patients are often unable to perform many activities of daily living. Many clinical measurements of breathlessness therefore quantify breathlessness in relation to the magnitude of the exertional task that evokes breathlessness. This approach relies on a patient's recall of daily tasks, ability to function or effort expended on different activities. There is also a complex interrelation between tasks that induce breathlessness, and those that are not possible due to breathlessness or are avoided because they cause breathlessness. Other types of indirect measures of breathlessness include breathlessness-related domains within quality of life instruments.

Medical Research Council Dyspnoea Scale

In use for several decades, the MRC Dyspnoea scale (Fletcher 1960) is the instrument most frequently used to assess what physical tasks induce breathlessness. It is a five-grade scale, ranging from 1 ('None' – 'Not troubled with breathlessness except with strenuous exercise') to 5 ('Very severe' – 'Too breathless to leave the house'). The patient chooses the most appropriate grade to describe their degree of breathlessness. It has proven to be a useful discriminative instrument for categorising patients according to the severity of their breathlessness, and has been shown to predict survival in patients with COPD (Celli et al. 2004).

The MRC Dyspnoea Scale has been shown to be too insensitive to detect small but potentially clinically relevant changes in breathlessness for individual patients. Therefore, it is not useful as an evaluative instrument to detect or measure change in response to an intervention. However, it does provide a useful baseline for initial assessment of a patient's limitations within the community setting. It is most useful as a technique to classify patients and to track disease trajectories over time. Because it primarily relates to the magnitude of task-induced breathlessness, there is no provision for assessment of associated effort, distress or quantification of breathlessness intensity.

The MRC Dyspnoea Scale has five grades as follows:

1: I only get breathless with strenuous exercise

2: I get short of breath when hurrying on the level or walking up a slight hill

3: I have to stop for breath when walking at my own pace on the level

4: I stop for breath after walking about 100 metres/yards or after a few minutes on the level

5: I am too breathless to leave the house or I am breathless when dressing or undressing.

The World Health Organisation functional classification for Pulmonary Hypertension (PH)

The World Health Organisation (WHO) and the New York Heart Association (NYHA) both provide similar four-point grading systems for functional limitation. The grades for these two measures are similar to the MRC in terms of the functional limitations denoted. However, the MRC scale is specifically focused on limitations due to breathlessness and not due to other symptoms, such as angina pain.

The WHO developed a system to help determine a patient's degree of limitation in their ability to do the activities of daily living. In general, the

WHO instrument is mainly used in pulmonary hypertension (PH). Patients with more severe PH tend to have a higher functional class. The four classes are as follows:

Class I: Patients with PH but without resulting limitation of physical activity. Ordinary physical activity does not cause undue dyspnoea of fatigue, chest pain or near syncope.

Class II: Patients with PH resulting in slight limitation of physical activity. They are comfortable at rest. Ordinary physical activity causes undue dyspnoea or fatigue, chest pain or near syncope.

Class III: Patients with PH resulting in marked limitation of physical activity. They are comfortable at rest. Less than ordinary activity causes undue dyspnoea or fatigue, chest pain or near syncope.

Class IV: Patients with PH with inability to carry out any physical activity without symptoms. These patients manifest signs of right heart failure. Dyspnoea and/or fatigue may even be present at rest. Discomfort is increased by any physical activity.

The New York Heart Association functional classification for heart failure

The New York Heart Association (NYHA) functional classification provides a simple way of classifying the extent of heart failure. It places patients in one of four categories, based on how much they are limited during physical activity, focusing on limitations/symptoms such as varying degrees of shortness of breath and/or angina pain.

The four classes are as follows:

Class I: No symptoms and no limitation in ordinary physical activity, such as shortness of breath when walking or climbing stairs.

Class II: Mild symptoms (such as mild shortness of breath and/or angina) and slight limitation during ordinary activity.

Class III: Marked limitation in activity due to symptoms, even during less than ordinary activity, such as walking short distances (20–100m). Only comfortable at rest.

Class IV: Severe limitations. Experiences symptoms even while at rest. Mostly applies to bedbound patients.

When reviewing a patient with PH or heart failure, there is likely to be documentation of their WHO or NYHA class in their case notes. As these instruments do not necessarily relate to breathlessness, it is recommended that the community practitioner use a breathlessness-specific questionnaire to ensure that this symptom is accurately captured.

Baseline Dyspnoea Index and Transitional Dyspnoea Index

The Baseline Dyspnoea Index (BDI) and Transitional Dyspnoea Index (TDI) (Mahler *et al.* 1984) were developed as a discriminative instrument. The BDI evaluates three dimensions: functional impairment, magnitude of effort and magnitude of task at a single time point. It rates the patient's breathlessness in each of these domains on a scale from 0 ('no impairment') to 4 ('severe impairment'). A companion scale, the Transitional Dyspnoea Index (TDI), is used to monitor changes from baseline over time and can be used to assess the impact of therapeutic interventions. The combined BDI/TDI was originally designed to be delivered by an experienced interviewer. More recently, a self-administered BDI/TDI version has been shown to correlate significantly with the interviewer-administered version (Mahler *et al.* 2004). As with the MRC scale, the BDI/TDI instruments are activity-determined and, although associated effort with specific tasks is included, there is no consideration of associated distress.

University of California–San Diego Shortness of Breath Questionnaire

Originally designed as a screening tool for pulmonary rehabilitation (Eakin *et al.* 1998), the University of California–San Diego Shortness of Breath Questionnaire (SOBQ) comprises 24 activity-related items that assess associated breathlessness over the preceding week. In addition, patients are requested to rate additional questions relating to fear of harm from over-exertion, and fear of shortness of breath. The SOBQ displays acceptable reliability taken over two days (r = 0.94) and good internal consistency (α = 0.91). Its validity has been demonstrated and is sensitive to improvements with rehabilitation (Meek & Lareau 2003). The instrument attempts to address aspects of affect denoted by perceived fear, though this is only in response to certain activities.

Pulmonary Functional Status and Dyspnoea Questionnaire

The Pulmonary Functional Status and Dyspnoea Questionnaire (PFSDQ) is a self-administered instrument rating breathlessness with 79 activities in six categories: self-care, mobility, eating, home management, social and recreational (Lareau *et al.* 1994). The instrument has since been modified and PFSDQ-M measures breathlessness associated with 10 activities and includes a fatigue component. Breathlessness is also measured as separate from activities with five items (Lareau *et al.* 1998). The PFSDQ-M is sensitive to small changes in breathlessness with activities, which make the instrument attractive for use within the community setting.

Measurement of breathlessness within quality of life scales

A number of questionnaires have been developed that evaluate the overall impact of cardio-pulmonary disease on a patient's quality of life. A well-designed measure of health-related quality of life should capture the pertinent and wide variety of consequences of a disease. Disease-specific quality of life questionnaires often have subscales, domains or components that assess the impact breathlessness may have on life quality. However, it is important to note that subscales may not have the same psychometric properties when used in isolation from the rest of the scale.

Chronic Respiratory Questionnaire

Guyatt and co-workers (1987) developed an interviewer-administered questionnaire, Chronic Respiratory Questionnaire (CRQ), comprising 20 items focusing on four dimensions of illness: breathlessness, fatigue, emotional functioning and the patient's feeling of control over the disease. A self-administered (self-report) version, the CRQ-SR, has since been developed (Schunemann *et al.* 2005). The CRQ and CRQ-SR have been extensively used and evaluated to measure quality of life in chronic respiratory and cardiac disease. The breathlessness component asks the patient to identify five activities that have induced a state of breathlessness within the last two weeks. Severity is evaluated on a 7-point scale. The breathlessness subscale can be considered on its own, though it is measured in terms of activity limitation and health-related quality of life.

St George's Respiratory Questionnaire

The St George's Respiratory Questionnaire (SGRQ) (Jones *et al.* 1992) is a self-administered 50-item questionnaire that measures three domains: symptoms, activity and impact of disease on daily life in COPD. The questionnaire has undergone refinement and the latest version (SGRQ-C) consists of 40 items (Meguro *et al.* 2007). Breathlessness is evaluated in terms of its impact on daily activities, for which there is a specific subscale called 'Activity'. It is also included in the 'Symptom' subscale, along with information relating to cough, sputum production and wheeze.

The SGRQ has also been used as a measure of quality of life for Interstitial Lung Disease (IPF). Since the SGRQ was not designed to measure health status in IPF, researchers have refined the instrument by identifying those items that were most reliable and valid for use in this population – SGRQ-I (Yorke *et al.* 2010b). The SGRQ-I consists of 34 items and has demonstrated good internal consistency and reliability of each component, and was comparable to the reliabilities for the corresponding components of the original SGRQ. Although the modified versions of the SGRQ contain fewer items, which enhances their clinical utility, a scoring algorithm is needed.

Chronic Obstructive Pulmonary Disease Assessment Test (CAT)

The CAT is a short (eight items, each on a five-point scale), simple questionnaire for assessing and monitoring COPD (Jones *et al.* 2009). It has good measurement properties and is sensitive to differences in health status. Although only one item refers to breathlessness, the CAT provides a quick and easy overall score for a patient's current health status. The CAT can be used in the community in an ongoing manner by comparing consecutive CAT scores for a patient with COPD, which helps with their long-term follow-up. CAT is easily available online at http://www.catestonline.co.uk

The Breathing Problems Questionnaire (BPQ)

The BPQ is a 13-domain QOL questionnaire for people with COPD (Hyland *et al.* 1994). A shorter version is also available and has demonstrated acceptable validity and reliability (Hyland *et al.* 1998). In a study that compared the BPQ-short version to the CRQ-short version, it was found that patients preferred the BPQ to the CRQ overall, and found it easier to complete (Best *et al.* 2009). This may be important when considering literacy levels and socioeconomic profiles of patients. It should therefore be considered more often as a self-complete HRQoL tool for patients with respiratory disease.

Chronic Heart Failure Questionnaire (CHQ)

The CHQ is a 20-item questionnaire, which was developed for use in CHF (Guyatt *et al.* 1989). It is a complex questionnaire to manage and it is administered by interview. It has three categories: dyspnoea, fatigue and emotional function. An increase in score shows an improvement in quality of life. This questionnaire was validated in a randomised, placebo-controlled trial of digoxin in CHF, and it was found to be most responsive to changes in dyspnoea and fatigue. The CHQ appears to be sensitive to patients with different severities of CHF.

Minnesota Living with Heart Failure Questionnaire (MLHFQ)

The MLHFQ was designed specifically for use in heart failure. It assesses the patient's perception of the physical, socioeconomic and psychological effects of CHF (Rector *et al.* 1987). Patients respond to 21 items using a six-point Likert scale (0–5). It is also possible to obtain subscale scores for physical and emotional domains. The questionnaire is easy to administer, short and easily understood. The measure has been found to be valid in comparison with other health outcome scales. It has been shown to discriminate between patients with CHF and those with symptomatic left ventricular dysfunction. It does not distinguish well between different severities of CHF. However, this is not an issue when measuring health status for a single individual.

Which is the most useful breathlessness questionnaire?

Many of the instruments discussed in this chapter were designed to be used as outcome measures in research. Questionnaires can also help clinicians to complete a thorough assessment but they need to be carefully selected to ensure that they are appropriate to specific patient groups and community settings. As demonstrated in this chapter, many tools are available. Some tools can be applied across different patient groups, whilst others have been developed for use in specific groups.

It is widely agreed that the most practical tool is the NRS. It can be used to directly assess breathlessness severity or distress, and it can be used in all patient groups. The NRS is quick and easy to apply, and patients can be encouraged to use it independently for self-monitoring. The Dyspnoea-12 has also been validated for use in a variety of conditions. It provides a simple assessment of both the physical and emotional consequences of living with breathlessness; this may help you identify which aspects of breathlessness management to focus on with a particular patient.

Summary

This chapter has discussed the clinical assessment of the breathless patient in the community. Regardless of underlying pathology, the assessment of breathlessness includes a clinical appraisal of the symptom and its severity. The person's reaction to breathlessness entails the measurement of different factors that may have an impact on their perception of breathlessness. Baseline assessment is essential in order to monitor any change in a patient's condition. Standardised questionnaires provide a method of carrying out ongoing monitoring of a patient in the community.

References

Abernethy, A.P. & Wheeler, J.L. (2008). Total dyspnoea. *Current Opinion and Supportive Palliative Care.* **2** (2), 110–13.

American Thoracic Society (ATS). (2012). Update on the mechanisms, assessment, and management of Dyspnoea. *American Journal of Respiratory Critical Care Medicine.* **185**, 435–52.

Bausewein, C., Farquhar, M., Booth, S., Gyles, M. & Higginson, I.J. (2007). Measurement of breathlessness in advanced disease: a systematic review. *Respiratory Medicine.* **101**, 399–410.

Best, H., Dyer, D. & Bott, J. (2009). Patient preferences for quality of life measures in pulmonary rehabilitation (PR): Breathing Problems Questionnaire Short Version (BPQ-SV) vs Chronic Respiratory Questionnaire Self-Report (CRQ-SR). *Thorax.* **64**, A97–A100.

Borg, G.A.V. (1982). Psychophysical bases of perceived exertion. *Medical Science and Sports Exercise.* **14**, 377.

Burdon, J.G., Juniper, E.F., Killian, K.J., Hargreave, F.E. & Campbell, E.J. (1982). The perception of breathlessness in asthma. *American Review of Respiratory Disease.* **126**(5) 825-8.

Caraceni, A. (2001). Evaluation and assessment of cancer pain and cancer pain treatment. *Acta Anaesthesiologica Scandinavica.* **45**, 1067–75.

Celli, B.R., Cote, C.G., Marin, J.M. & Casanova, C. (2004). The body-mass index, airflow obstruction, Dyspnoea, and exercise capacity index in Chronic Obstructive Pulmonary Disease. *New England Journal of Medicine.* **350** (10), 1005–12.

Cretikos, M.A., Bellomo, R., Hillman, K., Chen, J., Finfer, S. & Flabouris, A. (2008). Respiratory rate: the neglected vital sign. *The Medical Journal of Australia.* **188** (11) 657–9.

Dorman, S., Bryne, A. & Edwards, A. (2007). Which measurement scales should we use to measure breathlessness in palliative care? A systematic review. *Palliative Care.* **21**, 177–91.

Dowson, C.A., Kuijer, R.G. & Mulder, R.T. (2004). Anxiety and self management behaviour in chronic obstructive pulmonary disease: what has been learned? *Chronic Respiratory Disease.* **1**, 213–20.

Eakin, E.G., Resnikoff, P.M., Prewitt, L.M.,Ries, A.L. & Kaplan, R.M. (1998). Validation of a new dyspnea measure: the UCSD Shortness of Breath Questionnaire; University of California San Diego. *Chest.* **113**, 619-624.

Fletcher, C. (1960). Standardised questionnaire on respiratory symptoms: a statement prepared and approved by the MRC Committee on the aetiology of chronic bronchitis (MRC breathlessness score). *British Medical Journal.* **2**, 1665.

Gift, A.G. (1989). Validation of a vertical visual analogue scale as a measure of clinical dyspnoea. *Rehabilitation Nursing.* **14**, 323–5.

Guyatt, G.H., Berman, L.B., Townsend, M., Pugsley, S. & Chambers, L. (1987). A measure of quality of life for clinical trials in chronic lung disease. *Thorax.* **142**, 773–8.

Guyatt, G.H, Nogradi, S., Harlow, S., Sullivan, M. & Fallen, E. (1989). Development and testing of a new measure of health status for clinical trials in heart failure. *Journal of General Internal Medicine*. **4**, 101–7.

Hoogendoorn, M., Feenstra T.L., Hoogenveen, R.T. & Rutten-van Mölken, M.P.M.H. (2010). Long-term effectiveness and cost-effectiveness of smoking cessation interventions in patients with COPD. *Thorax*. **65**, 711–16

Hyland, M.E., Bott, J., Singh, S. & Kenyon, C.A. (1994). Domains, constructs and the development of the breathing problems questionnaire. *Quality of Life Research*. **3** (4), 245–56.

Hyland, M.E., Sing, S.J., Sodergren, S.C. & Morgan, M.P.L. (1998). Development of a shortened version of the breathing problems questionnaire suitable for use in a pulmonary rehabilitation clinic: A purpose-specific, disease-specific questionnaire. *Quality of Life Research*, **7** (3), 227–33.

Jones, P.W., Quirk, F.H., Baveystock, C.M. & Littlejohns, P. (1992). A self-complete measure of health status for chronic airflow limitation. The St. George's Respiratory Questionnaire. *American Review of Respiratory Disease*. **145** (6), 1321–7.

Jones, P.W., Harding, G., Berry, P., Wiklund, I., Chen, W.H. & Kline-Leidy, N. (2009). Development and first validation of the COPD Assessment Test. *European Respiratory Journal*. **34**, 648–54.

Kim, H.F.S., Kunik, M.E., Molinari, V.A., Hillman, S.L., Lalani, S., Orengo, C.A., Peterson, N.J., Nahas, Z. & Goodnight-White, S. (2000). Functional impairment in COPD patients: The impact of anxiety and depression. *Psychosomatics*. **41** (6), 465–71.

Lareau, S.C., Carrieri-Kohlman, V., Janson-Bjerklie, S. & Roos, P.J. (1994). Development and testing of the Pulmonary Functional Status and Dyspnoea Questionnaire (PFSDQ). *Heart Lung*. **23** (3), 242–50.

Lareau, S.C., Meek, P.M. & Roos, P.J. (1998). Development and testing of the modified version of the pulmonary functional status and Dyspnoea questionnaire (PFSDQ-M). *Heart and Lung*. **27** (3), 159–68.

Lavorini, F., Magnan, A., Dubus, J.C., Voshaar, T., Corbetta, L., Broeders, M., Dekhuijzen, R., Sanchis, J., Viejo, J.L., Barnes, P., Corrigan, C., Levy, M. & Crompton, G.K. (2008). Effect of incorrect use of dry powder inhalers on management of patients with asthma and COPD. *Respiratory Medicine*. **102** (4), 593–604.

Lundback, B., Lindberg, A. & Lindstrom, L. (2003). Not 15% but 50% of smokers develop COPD? Report from the Obstructive Lung Diseases in Northern Sweden Studies. *Respiratory Medicine*. **97**, 115–22.

Mahler, D.A. & Jones P.W. (1997). Measurement of dyspnea and quality of life in advanced lung disease. *Clinical in Chest Medicine*. **18** (3), 457-469.

Mahler, D.A., Weinberg, D.H., Wells, C.K. & Feinstein, A.R. (1984). The measurement of Dyspnoea. Contents, interobserver agreement, and physiologic correlates of two new clinical indexes. *Chest*. **85** (6), 751–8.

Mahler, D.A., Ward, J., Fierro-Carrion, G., Waterman, L.A., Lentine, T.F., Mejia-Alfaro, R. & Baird, J.C. (2004). Development of self-administered versions of modified baseline and transitional Dyspnoea indexes in COPD. *COPD*. **1**, 156–72.

Maurer, J., Rebbapragada, V., Borson, S., Goldstein, R., Kunik, M., Yohannes, A.M. & Hanania, N.A. (2008). Anxiety and depression in COPD. *Chest*. **134** (4 suppl), 43S–56S.

Meek, P. & Lareau, S.C. (2003). Critical outcomes in pulmonary rehabilitation: Assessment and evaluation of dyspnea and fatigue. *Journal of Rehabilitation Research and Development*. **40**(5), Supplement 2, 13–24.

Meguro, M., Barley, E.A., Spencer, S. & Jones, P.W. (2007). Development and validation of an improved, COPD-specific version of the St. George Respiratory Questionnaire. *Chest*. **132** (2), 456–63.

National Institute for Clinical Excellence (NICE). (2010). National Institute for Clinical Excellence COPD guidelines. http://www.nice.org.uk/nicemedia/live/13029/49397/49397.pdf. Accessed Online 13/02/2012.

O'Driscoll, B.R., Howard, L.S., Davidson, A.G, on behalf of the British Thoracic Society Oxygen Guidelines Development Group. (2008). Guidelines for the emergency use of oxygen in adult patients. *Thorax*. **63** (suppl 6).

Purdy, S., Griffin, T., Salisbury, C. & Sharp, D. (2011). Emergency respiratory admissions: influence of practice, population and hospital factors. *J. Health Serv. Res. Policy*. **16**(3): 133–40.

Rector, T., Kubo, S. & Cohen, J. (1987). Patients' self-assessment of their congestive heart failure: content, reliability and validity of a new measure – the Minnesota Living with Heart Failure Questionnaire. *Heart Failure*. **3**, 198–209.

Schünemann, H.J., Puhan, M., Goldstein, R., Jaeschke, R. & Guyatt, G. (2005). Measurement properties and interpretability of the Chronic Respiratory Disease Questionnaire (CRQ). *COPD: Journal of Chronic Obstructive Pulmonary Disease*. **2** (1), 81–89.

Swigris, J., Yorke, J., Sprunger, D., du Bois, R. & Fischer, A. (2010). The impact of dyspnoea on patients with connective tissue disease-related ILD. *Respiratory Medicine*. **104** (9), 1350–55.

Wilcock, A., Crosby, V., Clarke, D., & Tattersfield A., (1999). Repeatability of breathlessness measurements in cancer patients. *Thorax*, **54**, 375.

Yohannes, A.M., Willgoss, T.G., Baldwin, R.C. & Connolly, M.J. (2009). Depression and anxiety in chronic heart failure and chronic obstructive pulmonary disease: prevalence, relevance, clinical implications and management principles. *International Journal of Geriatric Psychiatry*. **25** (12), 1209–21.

Yorke, J., Moosavi, S., Shuldham, C. & Jones, P.W. (2010a). Quantification of dyspnoea using descriptors: Development and initial testing of the Dyspnoea-12. *Thorax*. **65** (1), 21–6.

Yorke, J., Jones, P.W. & Swigris, J. (2010b). Development and validity testing of an IPF-specific version of the SGRQ (the SGRQ-I). *Thorax*. **65**, 921–6.

4

Breathlessness and chronic obstructive pulmonary disease

Alison Newey and June Roberts

Patient perspective: Living with chronic obstructive pulmonary disease (COPD)

My name is Barbara, I am 69 years of age and I suffer from emphysema. I started with this illness in my early fifties; I had previously suffered with asthma. I was rather frightened when I was told of my illness – the thought of my lungs no longer working anywhere near like they should, the awful panic when you can't breathe properly. Ordinary little things seem twice as hard to do when you can't breathe; your life changes completely. I cried quite a lot in the early days of my illness when I was alone, mainly I think from frustration.

It is very hard accepting the change to your life, finding everything you do difficult. All your general jobs take longer and are sometimes quite painful. It's quite hard to cope with. Tiredness is one of the main things in my life now. I do get tired quite quickly.

Any jobs that need me to bend over (for example, cleaning the skirting boards or toilet, anything that is low down) make me very breathless and very uncomfortable. I have to stop for a break in between each job that I do.

I find breathing is hard work most of the time, except of course when I am sitting and relaxing. You find that you are up and down because you have left something behind and this causes a lot of breathlessness. It's the things you take for granted when you were well that take it out of you – for example, dressing and undressing, and shopping for clothes. Changing rooms are small and very hot so they are not really suitable for people with chest complaints.

When my illness took hold of me quite badly in 2012, I had a chest infection on my lungs; it took me a long time to get over that. My family were very protective, not wanting me to do too much or mix with people in shops or socially because of infection. But they have all realised that the more I do, the better it is for me. All my family are very supportive, especially my husband. I could never have coped without him. It was hard on my family because I was in and out of hospital all through 2010 and 2011. I have a very caring family.

I have had a new lease of life since I started going to pulmonary rehabilitation classes, which the COPD team recommended that I attend. The exercises are very good and have helped me to get on with my life a lot better and easier. I still get breathless of course but I have learned to cope with it much better.

Being breathless in public and coughing can be a little embarrassing but you just have to get on with it. I think people are becoming more aware of people with chronic illness now.

Breathlessness in COPD

At present, there is increasing pressure on healthcare services in the UK in relation to chronic illness. Planning of services requires reliable forecasting of the incidence of long-term conditions, and accurate estimation of the resources that can be provided within staffing and budgeting constraints. However, the true prevalence of COPD in England remains undetermined due to under-diagnosis of this long-term condition (DH 2010, NICE 2010).

Early signs of disease progression, such as coughing or shortness of breath on exertion, can easily be dismissed by the patient as being due to the effects of lifestyle or a lack of physical fitness. By the time that symptoms such as breathlessness become functionally limiting, the sufferer may already have a moderate to severe degree of damage to their lungs that cannot be repaired. Lung capacity will diminish naturally as a result of ageing but this calculated loss is accelerated by the inhalation of irritants that damage the physiological structure of the lungs. These irritants may include tobacco smoke and different types of dust to which people are exposed as a result of their occupation (GOLD 2011). Many people at risk of developing COPD could be screened in primary care and offered advice in an attempt to prevent them progressing to a more advanced stage of disease and disability.

This chapter looks at the background to a diagnosis of COPD, including a review of the causes of disease, its clinical features, diagnosis and assessment with a focus on breathlessness. In addition, COPD is compared to asthma, as these two presentations of lung disease are often poorly differentiated in primary care diagnoses.

Epidemiology

Around 835,000 people in England have been diagnosed with COPD, and an estimated 25,000–30,000 people die from COPD each year in Great Britain (Health and Safety Executive 2011). The number of people who suffer from a related disability is less defined because some individuals have not been formally diagnosed. Nevertheless a recent international survey of people with COPD aged between 45 and 67 indicated high societal and economic impact amongst working-age populations (Fletcher *et al.* 2011).

COPD is a progressive condition that is associated with lower socio-economic groups, particularly partially skilled and unskilled manual workers who are likely to have a history of smoking tobacco. However, these groups are also likely to demonstrate other variables that will impact upon their health and health behaviour, such as poor nutrition, poor education and poor housing (DH 2010, Points 26, 29). A combination of these social features can be a precursor for risk-taking behaviour, including smoking. Passive smoking is also a risk factor for COPD; people who are exposed to secondary, exhaled tobacco smoke at any age will be at risk of developing lung disease as a result (Jordan *et al.* 2011) (see Table 4.1). Although government directives have attempted to reduce the effects of poor health in disadvantaged groups and improve their access to healthcare services, around 2 million people may have undiagnosed COPD. Because the condition has not been diagnosed, these people do not realise that they are at risk of developing a severe long-term lung disorder.

Table 4.1: Risk factors for COPD

- Smoking tobacco
- Smoking cannabis
- Passive smoking
- Occupational exposure to dusts
- Domestic exposure to burning coal or wood

Pathophysiology

The symptoms of COPD stem from a chronic inflammatory response to inhaled tobacco smoke and other noxious particles that induce destruction of parenchymal lung tissue (resulting in emphysema) and narrowing of the small airways. Parenchymal destruction also leads to loss of alveolar attachment to the small airways, which decreases lung elastic recoil. This in turn diminishes the airways' ability to remain open during expiration. The mechanisms that lead to this amplified inflammatory response in COPD are not yet understood but may have an underlying genetic link, as for example in alpha 1 antitrypsin deficiency (Bourdin *et al.* 2009).

The structural changes caused by COPD lead to progressive airflow limitation, hyperinflation, air-trapping and reduced gas transfer, which induces progressive breathlessness. Hyperinflation reduces inspiratory capacity and increases functional residual capacity, particularly during activity. This is known as dynamic hyperinflation and it results in increased breathlessness during exercise. Hyperinflation is thought to develop early and is the main cause of exertional breathlessness (O'Donnell *et al.* 2001).

Although shortness of breath on exertion is the cardinal feature of COPD, people can also present with symptoms suggestive of chronic bronchitis – defined as the presence of cough and sputum for more than three months in two consecutive years. With these symptoms, the normal production of mucus is increased in response to the presence of inflammatory agents in the airways. This physiological reaction further contributes to structural airways changes and increases the incidence of respiratory infections (Donaldson & Wedzicha 2006).

Damage to the thin walls of the alveoli reduces the surface area available for gaseous exchange at the alveolar–capillary interface. Over time, this impaired function results in lower blood oxygen levels (hypoxaemia) and potentially a build-up of carbon dioxide (hypercapnia). As COPD progresses, hypoxic constriction of the pulmonary arteries and the loss of the alveolar capillary bed (due to emphysema) contribute to increased pressure in the pulmonary circulation, resulting in pulmonary hypertension. Progressive pulmonary hypertension can lead to right ventricular hypertrophy and right-sided heart failure, which in severe COPD is known as cor pulmonale (Bourdin *et al.* 2009).

Diagnosis and assessment in the community

The incidence of COPD is usually in the ≥35 years age group and may not be diagnosed until a stage of disease has been reached that is significant enough to necessitate a visit to the GP (DH 2010). In their seminal study of obstructive lung disease, Fletcher & Peto (1977) suggested that over 50% of lung capacity may have been lost by the time the patient seeks a medical review of their condition.

Diagnosis of COPD

The diagnosis of COPD is made on the basis of the clinical history, including the presence of predisposing risk factors, exclusion of alternative causes for symptoms, and physiological measurement of spirometry. These components collectively inform the clinician of a pattern of respiratory disease that is congruent with COPD.

According to NICE (2010), COPD is more likely in patients who are older than 35 and those who are smokers or ex-smokers.

NICE also lists signs or symptoms that may suggest COPD as:

- Breathlessness on exertion
- Chronic cough
- Regular sputum production
- Frequent episodes of bronchitis or chest infections
- Wheeze.

Diagnosis is made clearer if the patients do not have clinical features of other diseases, particularly asthma, and including bronchiectasis, congestive cardiac failure and lung cancer.

Spirometry

Improved recognition and care of patients with COPD is underpinned by high-quality, reliable, diagnostic spirometry, which is an important measure of lung volumes and **not to be confused with Peak Expiratory Flow Rate** which is a measure of the *rate* of airflow in L/min. The spirometry test is performed using a device called a spirometer, which comes in several different varieties. Spirometry is recommended for use in both the diagnosis and management of COPD in national guidelines and strategy (DH 2010, NICE 2010).

The significance of using spirometry to assess a respiratory disease is two-fold. The waveform and numerical values produced when a patient breathes into the spirometer give an indication of the respiratory diagnosis – for example, obstructive or restrictive patterns of lung disorder, and their severity. In COPD, an obstructed pattern of spirometry demonstrating post bronchodilator FEV_1/FVC ratio <0.7 supports the diagnosis. See Spirometry Readings Box below for a description of the different values obtained with spirometry testing and Table 4.2 for measuring severity of airflow obstruction using FEV1 in those with FEV_1/FVC ratio <0.7.

Spirometry readings

It is recommended that you consult a general respiratory textbook to become familiar with spirometry readings. Here are some basic definitions that may be helpful:

Forced Vital Capacity (FVC): the total volume of air that can be exhaled *forcibly* in one breath, following a maximum inspiration.

Forced Expired Volume in 1 second (FEV_1): the volume of the FVC that can be exhaled in the first second. You can expect a healthy person to force out at least 70% of their FVC in 1 second.

Vital Capacity (VC): (*slow or relaxed*), the total volume of air that can be exhaled in one breath without force following a maximum inspiration. Can identify air trapping – e.g. 'normal' other values but where symptoms may lead to suspicion of obstruction.

All expressed in litres and usually with % predicted – The test result as a percentage of the 'predicted values' or percentage of normal for people of similar characteristics (height, age, sex, race and weight).

FEV_1/ FVC (FER): ratio of FEV_1 to FVC: normal ≥0.7 or 70% (see Table 4.2 below for severity of airflow obstruction

Table 4.2: Measuring severity of airflow obstruction in COPD

In patient with FEV1/FVC ratio <0.7 post bronchodilator	
Severity	**FEV_1 % predicted**
Mild	≥80%
Moderate	50–79%
Severe	30–49%
Very severe	<30%

(Adapted from NICE 2010, GOLD 2011)

In COPD, the spirometric measurement of a forced exhalation does not change markedly after inhaling a bronchodilator. Although this feature is not exclusive to COPD, a careful clinical history in the context of the lung function results can aid diagnosis. Some patients with COPD may be under the impression that their respiratory diagnosis is asthma, although the presentation of this reversible lung disease differs from the clinical features of COPD. Where diagnostic uncertainty persists, an objective assessment of reversibility may be considered (NICE 2010). An accurate diagnosis is vital to ensure that the correct management strategy is applied. Table 4.3 (see page 62) highlights the clinical features that differentiate COPD from asthma.

Poorly performed spirometry and misinterpretation of the results can lead to misdiagnosis and inappropriate management. It is therefore essential that clinicians are trained and able to demonstrate competence to perform the test, identify errors and interpret results (Levy *et al.* 2009). There has been much debate about the quality and accuracy of primary care spirometry. However, if primary care practitioners are given adequate and appropriate training, they are able to obtain high-quality tests. According to Levy *et al.* (2009), the indications for spirometry in primary care are:

- Undiagnosed respiratory symptoms
- Suspected COPD
- Monitoring of established COPD
- Diagnosis of asthma.

Although there are no absolute contraindications to spirometry, there are some situations where it is advisable to delay testing or seek further advice from the local pulmonary function laboratory. Relative contraindications, according to Levy *et al.* (2009), include:

- Current or suspected respiratory infection
- Haemoptysis
- Recent myocardial infarction or pulmonary embolism
- Uncontrolled hypertension
- History of haemorrhagic cerebrovascular event
- Recent thoracic, abdominal or eye surgery
- Nausea, vomiting or pain
- Confusion and dementia.

Table 4.3: Clinical features differentiating COPD and asthma (NICE 2010)

Clinical features	COPD	Asthma
Smoker or ex-smoker	Nearly all	Possibly
Symptoms under age 35	Rare	Common
Chronic productive cough	Common	Uncommon
Breathlessness	Persistent and progressive	Variable
Night-time waking with breathlessness and/or wheeze	Uncommon	Common
Significant diurnal or day-to-day variability of symptoms	Uncommon	Common

Reflection point Reflection point Reflection point

Consider how the history and symptoms of COPD might differ from the clinical presentation of asthma.

Alpha 1 antitrypsin deficiency (AAT)

Alpha 1 antitrypsin deficiency is a rare genetic condition that leads to the early development of COPD. A detailed clinical history will highlight a background that is remarkable in the following respects:

- Presentation of symptoms at a younger age (<40 years of age)
- Non-smoker with no exposure to other risk factors
- Family history of similar clinical presentation
- Disproportionate level of breathlessness for history of exposure to risk factors.

This genetic predisposition to a severe form of COPD, a younger age of onset and fewer co-morbidities suggest that lung transplantation could be a treatment option for some patients. If AAT is suspected, community clinicians should therefore refer the patient for specialist assessment.

Assessment of the patient with COPD

It is important to note that the severity of airflow obstruction measured by FEV1% predicted correlates poorly with both symptoms and health-related quality of life (HRQL) (Jones 2011), and additional assessment is needed to capture the true impact of the disease on the individual (NICE 2010).

When assessing COPD beyond airflow obstruction, the aim is to determine the severity of the disease, its impact on HRQL and the risk of adverse outcomes such as hospital admission and death. NICE (2010) recommends that multidimensional assessment should therefore also include:

- Current level of symptoms, including breathlessness
- Exercise tolerance
- Exacerbation rate
- Presence of co-morbidities
- Body mass index
- Oxygen saturations.

Breathlessness

Progressive breathlessness is a cardinal symptom of COPD and a major cause of disability and anxiety. The questionnaires used to measure the direct and indirect impact of both breathlessness and COPD are discussed in Chapter 3, which explores the relative utility of the various instruments. A more detailed overview of the mechanisms of breathlessness and the individual nature of this symptom is provided in Chapter 2.

Chronic cough, sputum production and exacerbations

Patients with chronic cough and sputum production have an increased risk of exacerbations of COPD. In fact, the most reliable predictor of future exacerbations in an individual is their history of past exacerbations (Donaldson & Wedzicha 2006). An exacerbation of COPD is defined by GOLD (2011) as 'an acute event characterised by worsening of symptoms that is beyond day-to-day variations and leads to a change in medication'.

Exacerbations of COPD accelerate decline in lung function, resulting in increased breathlessness, reduced physical activity, reduced HRQL, increased risk of hospital admission and increased risk of death. The frequency and severity of exacerbations also increases as the COPD worsens; and most individuals do not return fully to pre-exacerbation levels of function. It is therefore important to monitor and record exacerbations in individual patients, and to target treatment and management so as to reduce the risk of repeated exacerbations in the future.

It has recently been shown that exacerbations occur across all severities of COPD, including mild disease (Hurst *et al.* 2010), and many patients are therefore likely to present to community clinicians for assessment and management. In an acute exacerbation, a patient is likely to present with the following:

- Breathlessness – described by the patient as being worse than usual day-to-day fluctuations
- Increased sputum purulence and volume
- Wheeze
- Chest tightness
- Reduced exercise tolerance.

Assessment of breathlessness is important, since it will direct the course of action required to treat the exacerbation and maintain the patient at home (NICE 2010). When there are signs of infection (such as excessive, purulent or green sputum), a short course of appropriate antibiotics can be prescribed. If the sputum remains clear or unchanged for that patient, antibiotics will not be required. Importantly, increased breathlessness or wheeze may indicate the need for a short course of oral steroids (NICE 2010).

All patients with chronic sputum production should be referred for physiotherapy to learn airway clearance techniques. This is a commonly forgotten therapy that can have a profound effect on the patient's ability to manage their symptoms (see Chapter 8 for further discussion of these techniques). Patients with chronic sputum production, if never taught to clear the excess secretions, will continue to suffer repeat exacerbations, as all the antibiotics and steroids on the planet wil not shift the actual mucus.

For those with chronic purulent or copious sputum production, a referral for further investigation of possible bronchiectasis is warranted.

Reflection point

Consider a patient who telephones to say that they are experiencing increased breathlessness. What initial questions will you ask the patient? Following this, you visit the patient at home to conduct a more thorough assessment. List the signs and symptoms that you would assess for, and what factors will help you to determine whether or not the patient is having an exacerbation of COPD, and whether the patient should be managed at home or in hospital.

Co-morbidities

As COPD often develops in long-term smokers, individuals frequently have other diseases related to smoking and ageing. However, the systemic effects of COPD (inflammation, hypoxia, poor diet and inactivity) may directly increase the risk of co-morbid disease. A recent analysis suggested that only 18% of people have COPD alone (Barnett *et al.* 2012). Co-morbidities are important because they increase the risk of hospitalisation and death for people with COPD. Co-morbidities that occur frequently in people with COPD include:

- Cardiovascular disease
- Heart failure
- Lung cancer
- Diabetes and metabolic syndrome
- Osteoporosis
- Depression and anxiety.

Because co-morbidity is so common in COPD (and can independently cause breathlessness and exercise limitation), differential diagnosis can often be difficult. It can also be challenging to correctly attribute symptoms and select appropriate treatment and management. For example, a patient with COPD, heart failure and anxiety could have increased breathlessness due to individual factors or a combination of components. In individual patients, the management of both COPD and co-morbidities should be optimised according to best practice guidelines. This includes the use of selective beta-blockers in ischaemic heart disease and heart failure where benefit outweighs potential risk (Salpeter *et al.* 2005). It is also important to actively look for co-morbidities in people with COPD – and to look for COPD in people with co-morbidities.

Depression and anxiety

Depression and anxiety are important co-morbidities because of their significant prevalence (particularly in people with more severe disease and in those experiencing exacerbations), and also because of their impact on outcomes such as hospitalisation. People with COPD are at risk of depression and anxiety due to progressive breathlessness and functional impairment. Poor recognition and lack of treatment in primary care can affect compliance with overall management, which may lead to increased unscheduled care utilisation. Screening tools, such as the Patient Health Questionnaire-2, can help clinicians recognise undiagnosed symptoms (Kroenke *et al.* 2003). Management options include pharmacotherapy, cognitive behavioural therapy and pulmonary rehabilitation (Maurer *et al.* 2008).

Reflection point Reflection point Reflection point

Consider the underlying pathophysiology of COPD. How might you distinguish between breathlessness that is related to COPD and breathlessness that is related to heart failure?

Treatment and management of COPD

Treatment and management of COPD should focus on control of symptoms and prevention of functional decline. Smoking cessation is the primary treatment, as it reduces lung function decline and symptoms. Smoking cessation therapy in COPD is extremely cost-effective and it is every healthcare professional's responsibility to help people give up smoking. In COPD, evidence-based stop smoking treatment consists of 90 minutes of intensive support plus pharmacotherapy with, for example, Nicotine Replacement Therapy, Bupropion or Varenicline (Hoogendoorn *et al.* 2010).

As we have seen, exacerbations of COPD have a significant adverse effect on symptoms, functional disability, healthcare utilisation and mortality. Influenza vaccination reduces exacerbation rates in people with COPD, and pneumococcal vaccination reduces the incidence of invasive pneumococcal disease. Vaccination with both may produce an additive effect that reduces exacerbations more effectively than either vaccine alone and is therefore recommended (NICE 2010).

Pharmacological therapy

Appropriate pharmacological treatment can reduce breathlessness, the frequency and severity of exacerbations, and improve health status and exercise tolerance. However, to date, none of the existing medications for COPD has been conclusively shown to modify long-term decline in lung function (NICE 2010, GOLD 2011).

Inhaled bronchodilators are the cornerstone of treatment in COPD because they reduce air trapping and dynamic hyperinflation, thus reducing breathlessness and improving exercise capacity (O'Donnell *et al.* 2001). The extent of improvement is not predictable from improvements in the FEV1. Bronchodilators should therefore be given as needed or regularly to prevent or improve symptoms. Long-acting bronchodilators are more effective for maintaining relief from breathlessness than short-acting agents. Long-acting beta 2 agonists (LABA) and long-acting anti-muscarinic agents (LAMA) bronchodilators improve HRQL, and reduce exacerbation rate and hospitalisations. LAMA has additional evidence that also supports improvements in the effectiveness of pulmonary rehabilitation (Kesten *et al.* 2008).

The addition of regular treatment with combination inhaled corticosteroid/LABA is indicated in more severe disease (FEV1 $<50\%$), when breathlessness is not controlled with LABA and/or LAMA alone, or in those with FEV1 $>50\%$, particularly when exacerbations are a feature. Oral corticosteroids are only indicated for the treatment of exacerbations of COPD where they have been found to reduce the severity and duration of the episode (NICE 2010, GOLD 2011). For some patients, difficulties with sputum clearance can increase breathlessness. The addition of mucolytic and nebulised therapies may ease expectoration, in combination with sputum clearance techniques.

Theophylline can be trialled (with caution due to its adverse side effect profile), but only if inhaled long-acting bronchodilators are ineffective or not tolerated. High dose nebulised bronchodilators may also be considered in patients with distressing or disabling breathlessness despite maximal inhaled therapy. However, they should not be prescribed without assessment of the patients'/carers' ability to use the equipment and assessment of evidence of benefit. In very severe disease, where breathlessness remains unrelieved by conventional COPD treatments, opioids can be used to palliate symptoms. Benzodiazepines and major tranquilisers can also be trialled although there is limited evidence to support their use in COPD (NICE 2010, GOLD 2012).

Non-pharmacological therapy

Recognising the end of life in people with COPD is difficult, and it has been argued that reliance on prognostic indicators and Gold Standard Framework (GSF) registers leads to delay in the optimal management of breathlessness for this group of patients (Pinnock *et al.* 2011). It is therefore important that community clinicians think beyond traditional pharmacological disease treatment regimes and consider additional interventions to relieve this distressing symptom. Non-pharmacological techniques, such as breathing control and pacing, may be particularly helpful. Additional information on non-pharmacological interventions and managing breathlessness at the end of life can be found in Chapters 8 and 10.

Oxygen

Oxygen is a treatment for hypoxaemia (not breathlessness). In COPD, it can be a lifesaver for some and a killer for others. In people with hypoxaemic COPD, treatment with long-term oxygen therapy (LTOT) reduces mortality, improves symptoms and enhances quality of life (Medical Research Council Working Party 1981). However, oxygen must be introduced cautiously because people with COPD are also at risk of increased sensitivity to the effects of supplemental oxygen. In this group of patients, there is a potential loss of hypoxic respiratory drive and a high risk of carbon dioxide retention, leading to type II respiratory failure. Specialist assessment is therefore recommended before oxygen is introduced (PCC 2011).

Whilst there is good evidence for the use of LTOT in hypoxaemic COPD, there is no benefit from short burst oxygen (SBOT) in non-hypoxaemic patients. Furthermore, although ambulatory oxygen can reduce breathlessness during activity, it too should only be prescribed after careful assessment to those who desaturate on exercise, or as a supplement to LTOT for people who are prepared to use oxygen to get out of the house (NICE 2010, GOLD 2011, PCC 2011). The patient may require two different oxygen prescriptions: a resting one (for example, for sitting and sleeping); and one for ambulatory use (for example, for walking, exercising and performing activities of daily living). Even in palliative situations, oxygen only appears to benefit those who are hypoxaemic; less burdensome solutions to relieve breathlessness should be considered in non-hypoxaemic patients (Abernethy *et al.* 2010).

It is therefore recommended that clinicians monitor pulse oximetry when assessing people with COPD at least annually and more often in those with more severe disease. When stable, patients with oxygen saturations persistently ≤92% should be referred to a specialist for blood gas analysis and assessment for appropriate oxygen prescription (NICE 2010, GOLD 2011). There is also significant risk of harm if supplemental oxygen is given unnecessarily or at too high a level during exacerbations of COPD. In these situations, oxygen (if required) should be titrated to maintain a target saturation of 88–92% (O'Driscoll *et al.* 2008). Once stable, the patient's need for oxygen should be reassessed after about six weeks if saturations remain ≤92% (NICE 2010).

Many patients with normal oxygen saturations have been incorrectly prescribed oxygen because they suffer from breathlessness. Once prescribed, it can be difficult to remove, even when it is clear that it provides no clinical benefit. Home oxygen therapy is provided to about 85,000 people in England at a cost of approximately £110 million a year; yet it is estimated that around 30% of people either derive no clinical benefit from it or do not use it as prescribed. This is important, as oxygen equipment (whether used or unused) costs the NHS a great deal (PCC 2011). Community clinicians should therefore be alert to the risks and costs associated with non-specialist oxygen prescribing.

Pulmonary rehabilitation

The most important non-pharmacological intervention in the management of COPD is pulmonary rehabilitation (PR). Formal PR restores function through a programme of individualised tailored exercise training, alongside education and support designed to encourage long-term behaviour change (IMPRESS 2011). Courses usually consist of at least two supervised sessions a week for around six weeks.

The benefits of PR include reduced breathlessness, increased exercise capacity, improved psychological wellbeing and enhanced HRQL (NICE 2010). Up to 50% of people who attend PR will show highly significant improvements in breathlessness, fatigue, and mastery of their condition (Griffiths *et al.* 2001).

PR offered post exacerbation also reduces hospital attendance and mortality (Puhan *et al.* 2011) and is cost effective (Griffiths *et al.* 2001). Because of these important health gains, clinicians should actively seek out those who would benefit from PR, encourage acceptance for referral and support attendance (NICE 2010, GOLD 2011). Patients with MRC ≥3, or people who consider themselves disabled by their breathlessness or who have had hospital admissions should be offered PR. As the evidence for benefit from formal PR is not yet established for less symptomatic patients, those with MRC ≤2 should be encouraged to exercise and stay active to help prevent functional decline (IMPRESS 2011). For those patients who desaturate on exercise and who have demonstrated an improvement with supplemental oxygen at assessment, the use of ambulatory oxygen can significantly increase the benefit of PR – by up to 120% (Dyer *et al.* 2012).

PR should be viewed as a fundamental treatment for COPD, rather than an optional extra. Yet people with COPD who have breathlessness and exercise limitation may have difficulty understanding why they should be referred for exercise training. Addressing patient concern about PR can improve uptake and completion rates (Harris *et al.* 2008). The decision to refer should therefore be used as an opportunity to explore the patient's understanding of PR, address concerns and educate them about the benefits of attending a PR programme. The improvements gained through PR fade over time. A repeat programme is likely to be of benefit if the last completed course was one year ago or earlier, where there is accelerated functional decline or following a hospital admission. All individuals who complete a course of pulmonary rehabilitation should be supported to continue exercising.

Summary

This chapter has reviewed the background to a diagnosis of COPD and the risk factors that may impact upon this long-term condition. Treatment is aimed at maintaining lung capacity and managing symptoms as they arise. Although COPD cannot be cured, there is value in optimising therapy, particularly in encouraging participation in PR, to enable the patient to be active and feel confident about managing their symptoms.

References

Abernethy, A., McDonald, C.F., Frith, P.A., Clark, K. & Herndon, J.E. (2010). Effect of palliative oxygen versus room air in relief of breathlessness in patients with refractory Dyspnoea: a double blind, randomized controlled trial. *The Lancet*. **376** (9743), 784–93.

Barnett, K., Mercer, S.W., Norbury, M., Watt, G., Wyke, S. & Guthrie, B. (2012). Epidemiology of multimorbidity and implications for health care, research, and medical education: a cross-sectional study. *The Lancet*. Published online 10 May 2012. DOI:10.1016/S0140-6736(12)60240-2.

Bourdin, A., Burgel, P-R, Chanez, P., Garcia, G., Perez, T. & Roche, N. (2009). Recent advances in COPD: pathophysiology, respiratory physiology and clinical aspects, including comorbidities. *European Respiratory Review*. **18** (114), 198–212.

Department of Health (DH). (2010). Strategy for services for Chronic Obstructive Pulmonary Disease (COPD) in England – consultation document.

Donaldson, G.C. & Wedzicha, J.A. (2006). COPD exacerbations. 1: Epidemiology. *Thorax*. **61**, 164–68.

Dyer, F., Callaghan, J., Cheema, K. & Bott, J. (2012). Ambulatory oxygen improves the effectiveness of pulmonary rehabilitation in selected patients with chronic obstructive pulmonary disease. *Chronic Respiratory Disease*. **9** (2), 83–91.

Fletcher, C. & Peto, R. (1977). The natural history of chronic airflow obstruction. *British Medical Journal*. **1** (6077), 1645–48.

Fletcher, M., Upton, J., Taylor-Fishwick, J., Buist, S.A., Jenkins, J., Hutton, J., Barnes, N., Van Der Molan, T., Walsh, J.W., Jones, P.W. & Walker, S. (2011). COPD uncovered: an international survey on the impact of chronic obstructive pulmonary disease [COPD] on a working age population. *BMC Public Health*. **11**, 612.

Global Initiative for Chronic Obstructive Lung Disease (GOLD). (2011). http://www.goldcopd.org/uploads/users/files/GOLD_PocketGuide_2011_Jan18.pdf. Accessed online 17/02/2012.

Griffiths, T.L., Phillips, C.J., Davies, S., Burr, M.L. & Campbell, I.A. (2001). Cost effectiveness of an outpatient multidisciplinary pulmonary rehabilitation program. *Thorax*. 56, 779–784

Health & Safety Executive (2011). Chronic Obstructive Pulmonary Disease (COPD) in Great Britain. http://www.hse.gov.uk/statistics/causdis/copd/copd.pdf. Accessed online 20/02/2012.

Harris, D., Hayter, M. & Allender, S. (2008), Improving the uptake of pulmonary rehabilitation in patients with COPD: qualitative study of experiences and attitudes. *British Journal General Practice*. **58**, 703–10.

Hoogendoorn, M., Feenstra, T.K., & Hoogenveen, R.T. (2010). Long term effectiveness and cost effectiveness of smoking cessation interventions in COPD. *Thorax*. **65**: 711–18

Hurst, J.R., Vestbo, J., Anzueto, A., Locantore, N., Mullerova, H. for the Evaluation of COPD Longitudinally to Identify Predictive Surrogate Endpoints (ECLIPSE) Investigators (2010). Susceptibility to Exacerbation in Chronic Obstructive Pulmonary Disease. *New Eng J Med*. **636**, 1128–38.

IMPRESS (2011) Guide to Pulmonary Rehabilitation http://www.impressresp.com/index.php?option=com_docman&task=doc_view&gid=41&Itemid=82 Accessed online 4/1/13.

Jones, P. (2011). Functional status, health status and primary care. *Primary Care Respiratory Journal*. **20** (3), 227–28.

Jordan, R.E., Cheng, K.K., Miller, M.R. & Abab, P. (2011). Passive smoking and chronic obstructive pulmonary disease: cross-sectional analysis of data from the Health Survey for England. *BMJ Open*2011;**1**:e000153 doi:10.1136/bmjopen-2011-000153.

Kesten, S., Casaburi, R., Kukafka, D. & Cooper, C.B. (2008). Improvement in self-reported exercise participation with the combination of tiotropium and rehabilitative exercise training in COPD patients. *International Journal of Chronic Obstructive Pulmonary Disease* **3**, 127–36.

Kroenke, K., Spitzer, R.L. & Williams, J.B. (2003). The Patient Health Questionnaire-2: validity of a two-item depression screener. *Medical Care* **41**(11), 1284–92.

Levy, M.L., Quanjer, P.H., Booker, R., Cooper, B.G., Holmes S. & Small I.R. (2009) Diagnostic spirometry in primary care: Proposed standards for general practice compliant with American Thoracic Society and European Respiratory Society recommendations. *Primary Care Respiratory Journal.* **18**(3), 130–47.

Maurer, J., Rebbapragada, V., Borson, S., *et al.* (2008). Anxiety and depression in COPD: current understanding, unanswered questions, and research needs. *Chest* **134**(4 Suppl):43S–56S.

Medical Research Council Working Party (1981) Long term domiciliary oxygen therapy in chronic hypoxic cor pulmonale complicating chronic bronchitis and emphysema. *Lancet.* **I**, 681–86.

National Institute for Clinical Excellence (NICE). (2010). National Institute for Clinical Excellence COPD guidelines. http://www.nice.org.uk/nicemedia/live/13029/49397/49397.pdf. Accessed online 13/02/2012.

O'Donnell D.E., Revill, S.M. & Webb, K.A. (2001) Dynamic hyperinflation and exercise intolerance in Chronic Obstructive Pulmonary Disease. *American Journal of Respiratory and Critical Care Medicine.* **164**, 770–77.

O'Driscoll, B.R., Howard, L.S. & Davidson, A.G, on behalf of the British Thoracic Society Oxygen Guidelines Development Group. (2008). Guidelines for the emergency use of oxygen in adult patients. *Thorax* **63** (suppl 6).

Pinnock, H., Kendall, M., Murray S.A., Levack, P., Porter, M. & Macknee, W. (2011) Living and dying with severe chronic obstructive pulmonary disease: multi-perspective longitudinal qualitative study. *BMJ.* **342**, d142.

Primary Care Commissioning (PCC) (2011) Home Oxygen Service Assessment and Review: Good practice guide http://www.improvement.nhs.uk/lung/GoodPracticeGuides/Homeoxygenservice/tabid/193/Default.aspx Accessed online 4/1/13.

Puhan, M.A., Gimeno-Santos, E., Scharplatz, M., Troosters, T., Walters, E.H. & Steurer, J. (2011). Pulmonary rehabilitation following exacerbations of chronic obstructive pulmonary disease. *Cochrane Database of Systematic Reviews* **10**.

Salpeter, S., Ormiston, T. & Salpeter, E. (2005). Cardioselective beta-blockers for chronic obstructive pulmonary disease. *Cochrane Database of Systematic Reviews* 2005:CD003566.

5

Breathlessness and heart failure

Miriam Johnson and Amy Gadoud

Patient perspective: Living with heart failure

My name is George and I am 85 years old. Since I retired from my job as a transport manager, I have had two heart attacks. I was not aware of the first one – it was only discovered after my GP sent me for some tests. The tests showed it had not left any scars but that one-third of my heart was not working. I later had a second heart attack and I was admitted to hospital and kept in for six days. I have gradually got worse with my breathing over the last few years, and I have now been diagnosed with heart failure and have support from the nurse specialist and consultant who work with my GP.

My job was very stressful, with long hours, but I was always very fit. I used to play football and cricket and enjoyed going to shows and dancing. We saw all the big American stars, including Frank Sinatra. I never smoked so it was a bit of a shock to have a heart attack. Now I can only walk 20 yards on the flat before I have to stop to catch my breath. On the slightest incline, I am extremely short of breath after just a few steps. I struggle to get off the settee and easy-chair without assistance. I find it difficult to bend and pick anything up off the floor. Although I attended cardiac rehabilitation after my heart attacks, I do not think I could do it now.

The consultant tried some new tablets, which unfortunately did not agree with me. They made my blood pressure very low, causing me to have blackouts. I was admitted to hospital for a few days because one of the blackouts caused me to fall in the bathroom and I crushed one of my vertebrae. The tablets have been stopped and I have not had any more blackouts. I find it difficult to attend hospital and GP appointments. The walk from the car park is too much and there is never a disabled space. Next week I am having a heart scan and will get a taxi there and back – it is easier.

I do find that I get annoyed because of my breathing and I am probably at my worst now. I just have to live with it. I struggle with most things at home and have to rely on my wife to help. She does 99% of everything. I can just about manage to get washed and dressed – but bending down, to put my socks and shoes on, makes me really breathless. I cannot shower myself, as I can't get my arms up, but just about manage to have a bath. Sometimes it is just too much and I have a wash instead. I can get a bit depressed and frustrated because I can't do things. It can also get a bit frightening when I can't catch my breath.

I do feel reassured by my nurse who visits me at home. She gets me to weigh myself every morning. Fortunately, my weight is quite static. I also have oxygen now and I find that can help. I want to thank all the hospital staff and particularly my wife, who has been a tower of strength even though she is not very well herself.

Breathlessness in heart failure

Chronic heart failure (CHF) is a common final pathway for many cardiac diseases, the most prevalent in Western society being ischaemic heart disease, followed by hypertensive heart disease. CHF is therefore an escalating and major public health concern. Although the true incidence is not increasing, this age-related disease has become more prevalent, because more people are living into old age. This means that many patients are living with this condition in the community.

In addition to the growing elderly population, more people survive acute coronary artery disease and thus live to develop CHF. As the treatment of CHF has improved so dramatically over the past two decades, many more live to a progressive end-stage CHF. As CHF is largely a disease of the elderly, patients often have significant co-morbidities contributing to their symptom burden. These may include, for example, renal disease, chronic obstructive pulmonary disease (COPD) and diabetes, which also have an impact on survival.

Chronic heart failure is a clinical syndrome described as the inability of the heart to pump an adequate amount of oxygenated blood to meet the body's demands (adequate cardiac output). It is a condition that is marked by shortness of breath (at rest or during exertion), fatigue, and signs of fluid retention such as pulmonary congestion or ankle swelling, and evidence of abnormal structure or function of the heart. Abnormal sodium levels and fluid retention (overload) are also often present with congestive heart failure.

Pathophysiology of heart failure due to left ventricular dysfunction

In CHF, when the heart has been damaged, there are often changes in its size, shape, structure and function which impair the left ventricular function. This results in a fall in cardiac output, which leads to the activation of several compensatory mechanisms (sympathetic nervous system, renin-angiotensin-aldosterone system, ventricular dilation and ventricular hypertrophy), all of which aim to restore adequate left ventricular function.

Two key interlinking models, which explain the downward spiral of untreated chronic heart failure, have usefully guided the development of targeted therapy that can stabilise the disease for many patients for a significant length of time (George & Linda 2001).

The neurohormonal model describes the activation of the renin-angiotensin system as a result of poor renal perfusion pressure, and in turn the stimulation of the sympathetic nervous system (Packer 1992). This understanding has led to the highly effective triple therapy of angiotensin-converting enzyme inhibitor, beta blocker and aldosterone antagonist agents.

The peripheral model describes the pathological changes in skeletal muscle due to poor perfusion, neurohormonal and cytokine activation and lack of fitness. This myopathy is a cause of fatigue and breathlessness. Interventions to preserve or improve muscle function are therefore also important in managing CHF and its key symptoms (Clark *et al.* 1996).

Reflection point

Revision of the neurohormonal pathophysiology of heart failure helps explain how the key medications work to reduce the downward spiral of worsening heart failure.

Causes of congestive heart failure

There are thought to be many factors in the development of congestive heart failure. Common causes (either alone or in combination) are listed below:

- Ischaemic heart disease
- Hypertensive heart disease
- Valvular heart disease
- Cardiomyopathy (viral, toxic, e.g. alcohol)
- Dysrhythmias
- Pericardial disease
- Congenital heart disease.

General disease assessment and management

Functional CHF classification

The New York Heart Association (Criteria Committee of the New York Heart Association, 1994) has published a 'functional' classification for congestive heart failure, consisting of four classes:

Table 5.1: NYHA functional classification

NYHA class	Symptoms
I	No symptoms and not limited by ordinary physical activity, e.g. shortness of breath when walking, climbing stairs, etc.
II	Mild symptoms (mild shortness of breath and/or angina), leading to slight limitation during ordinary activity
III	Marked limitation in activity due to symptoms, even during less-than-ordinary activity, e.g. walking short distances (20–100m); comfortable only at rest
IV	Severe limitations. Experiences symptoms even while at rest.

The NYHA classification enables ongoing assessments to be made, based on the patient's subjective experience of symptoms.

Exacerbations of CHF may be florid and easily diagnosed – for example, acute pulmonary oedema. However, the symptoms and clinical signs of heart failure are often non-specific, and more specific signs (such as raised jugular venous pressure or third heart sound) are not present in every patient with heart failure. Therefore, a high clinical index of suspicion and careful history and examination is needed to confirm the diagnosis, to identify precipitating factors and co-morbid conditions so that appropriate management can be planned for each individual (NICE 2010). Community assessment includes deciding whether the patient can be appropriately managed at home or requires hospital admission. A detailed discussion of disease assessment is beyond the scope of this book. Here, the focus is on the symptom of breathlessness, for which a full holistic assessment of 'total-breathlessness' is needed, and this is described in more detail in Chapter 3.

Optimal management of CHF includes up-titration of angiotensin-converting enzyme inhibitor, beta blocker and aldosterone antagonist agents to maximal tolerated dose or until the target dose has been reached. Patients will usually need loop diuretics to help manage fluid overload – sometimes by parenteral administration if the gut has become too oedematous to allow oral absorption. In addition, attention to managing rhythm disturbance (for example, by controlling the ventricular rate in atrial fibrillation) may help maximise the residual function.

The introduction of cardiac devices has added another management layer. For patients with cardiac asynchrony, even those who are significantly symptomatic (NYHA III in Table 5.1 above), cardiac resynchronisation therapy (CRT) may provide both symptom and survival benefit (Reviriego 2011). CRT allows sequential contraction of the right and left ventricle to enable maximal possible ejection fraction. The CRT device may also have a cardiac defibrillator function (CRT-ICD), which prevents sudden cardiac death due to arrhythmias. However, there is little evidence that survival is increased if this device is placed in a person with NYHA IV disease.

Finally, there are the options of left ventricular assist device (LVAD) therapy and cardiac transplantation. Initially, an LVAD was only used as a bridge to an expected recovery (for example, in acute viral myocarditis) and definitive intervention (cardiac transplantation). But LVADs are now being used as a 'destination therapy', sometimes remaining in situ in patients indefinitely. For the majority of patients, complex treatment (such as a transplant or an LVAD) is not an option. Only about 4000 heart transplants are carried out annually worldwide (Pitsis 2008).

Daily management at home centres upon patient self-management programmes, ideally supported by a heart failure nurse specialist and increasingly with remote telemonitoring of weight and vital signs. Patients are taught to weigh themselves at the same time every day and to increase the dose of loop diuretic if they have put weight on, according to a written algorithm. The aim is to prevent hospital admission for fluid overload by addressing any problem early enough to manage with oral medication.

Breathlessness in CHF

Breathlessness is a cardinal symptom in CHF and contributes to the basis of the NYHA classification of disease severity. Breathlessness is also a feature of co-morbid COPD. Management programmes (including exercise) may be limited by other co-morbid conditions such as arthritis. Thus the breathless patient with CHF should be considered within the context of other illnesses that may also be present. Although much of the research on interventions for the management of breathlessness has been conducted in people with COPD or cancer, the generic principles can be applied to chronic breathlessness due to any cause.

Breathlessness due to cancer or COPD tends to worsen in the months before death but in CHF this severity trajectory is less clear. For many patients, it is chaotic, reflecting the periods of stability and unpredictable decompensations of the CHF itself (Currow *et al.* 2010). However, the concept of 'total-breathlessness' applies to shortness of breath from any aetiology, with contributing physical, psychological, financial, social and spiritual factors (Abernethy & Wheeler 2008).

Reflection point Reflection point Reflection point

Does the 'total-breathlessness model' alter the way you take a history from a patient with breathlessness? What new areas might you explore?

Mechanisms of breathlessness

The mechanisms involved in the perception of breathlessness are complex (see Chapter 2), and it is likely that these all play a role in people with

CHF. Nevertheless, there are certain features of CHF that should be noted with regard to the perception of breathlessness. Traditionally, shortness of breath in CHF was thought to be caused by simple abnormalities in central haemodynamics: 'backward' failure, leading to a rise in pulmonary venous pressure, with stiff or even oedematous lungs resulting in breathlessness. However, exercise limitation is not directly related to the severity of abnormal central haemodynamics (Harrington, Anker & Coats 2001).

In addition, people with CHF demonstrate an excessive ventilatory pattern in response to exercise despite, rather surprisingly, better than normal arterial blood gases during exercise. This drive to excessive ventilatory response is thought to arise from enhanced chemoreflexes, and the skeletal myopathy, which causes an enhanced ergoreflex. The ergoreflex is a neurally mediated response to exercise, in proportion to the amount of exercise but in inverse proportion to the volume of skeletal muscle. For example, smaller muscles (as in the arm) induce a greater response to exercise than larger muscles in the legs. Stimulation of the ergoreflex stimulates the sympathetic nervous system and the ventilatory response. The ergoreflex theory explains the two key symptoms of CHF – breathlessness and fatigue – and underlines the importance of interventions designed to maintain muscle bulk and function. Other factors may also be at play, but these two (enhanced chemo and ergoreflexes) appear to be major drivers for CHF-related breathlessness and fatigue (Clark *et al* 1996; Packer 1992).

Management of breathlessness in CHF

In keeping with the concept of 'total-breathlessness', management of CHF-related breathlessness in the community starts with a full holistic assessment. In this holistic assessment, the patients' and carers' need for information and communication is often overlooked. Many patients do not even know their diagnosis and this results in poor understanding, lack of compliance with treatment and less control over their management of their condition (Banerjee *et al.* 2010).

Optimisation of the underlying disease should include, for example, ensuring that the patient is titrated to maximally tolerated heart failure medication, taking into account any co-morbidities (including psychological co-morbidities such as anxiety and depression). Careful attention should be paid to potentially reversible causes of shortness of breath. Clinical assessment of fluid status is important, with attention paid to increased weight, a raised jugular venous pressure and oedema. Titration of diuretics to gain fluid balance is a first step in the management of breathlessness due to decompensated fluid overload

It is also important to distinguish between breathlessness, particularly at night (due to fluid overload, leading to paroxysmal nocturnal dyspnoea), and distressed arousal following an episode of obstructive or central sleep apnoea (due to sleep-disordered breathing). Breathlessness due to fluid overload is managed by restoring fluid balance through the use of diuretics, while management of breathlessness as a result of sleep apnoea includes continuous positive airways pressure or oxygen therapy at night.

Reflection point

Recognition of common reversible causes of breathlessness is a vital first step in the management of breathlessness. In a patient with heart failure, what might some of these causal factors be?

A particular challenge is coordination of care between professionals, especially between primary and secondary care, in the management of breathlessness in heart failure. Medication may be appropriately stopped during an inpatient exacerbation but may then need to be reintroduced or up-titrated in the community. Several conversations about the disease and its management, including self-management, may be required. This is where a good community team can have a key role.

The rest of this chapter will focus on situations where these stages of management have already taken place but the symptom of refractory breathlessness remains.

Non-pharmacological management

Cardiac rehabilitation generally includes exercise programmes as well as educational and psychological support. In 2009, a Cochrane review of 29 randomised controlled trials (RCTs) of exercise-based interventions in people with CHF showed that patients receiving exercise improved in exercise ability, oxygen utilisation in six-minute walk tests, and general quality of life (Rees *et al.* 2009).

Mindfulness–based stress reduction (MBSR) is another non-pharmacological technique used in chronic illnesses, usually delivered as an eight-week programme. A cohort study of 208 people with CHF were randomised to receive MBSR in addition to usual care for eight weeks or usual care only with follow-up for one year (Sullivan *et al.* 2009). Improvement was demonstrated in the MBSR group at 12 months. Anxiety and depression scores both went down over time. As anxiety and breathlessness seem to be closely linked, MBSR techniques may be helpful as part of an overall management plan for breathlessness. A well-conducted systematic review of non-exercise, non-pharmacological management of breathlessness, concluded that there is a big gap in the evidence outside of COPD (Bausewein *et al.* 2008). Recommendations were therefore extrapolated from the studies on COPD. There were three studies looking at patients with CHF. One study included participants with different diagnoses (some with CHF) demonstrating a reduced sensation of breathlessness with a hand-held fan (Galbraith *et al.* 2010). The other two studies were confined to patients with CHF. Goodyer *et al.* 1995 in an RCT of a patient medical counselling programme showed a reduction in breathlessness intensity, measured by 0–100mm visual analogue scale. An RCT of a muscle relaxation training programme showed improvement in psychological distress but the change in symptom status was non significant (Yu *et al.* 2007)

Pharmacological management

There are similar difficulties in assessing pharmacological management, and very few studies involving participants with CHF. A Cochrane review of opioids for the relief of breathlessness due to different aetiologies concluded that there was evidence of benefit (Jennings *et al.* 2002) but the trials were small, and only one of them included people with CHF. After the Cochrane review, a pilot study of 10 people with CHF demonstrated relief of breathlessness with four days' morphine, compared with a placebo (Johnson *et al.* 2002). Yet a subsequent, adequately powered study, comparing oxycodone, morphine and placebo in a similar population, failed to show benefit from either opioid after four days' administration (Oxberry *et al.* 2011). Interestingly, a three month open label follow up study of those who chose to continue an opioid or not showed a statistically significant improvement in breathlessness in those who continued an opioid (Oxberry *et al.* 2013). Although this is only preliminary data, it suggest that opioids should be given a therapeutic trial in people with heart failure for more than 4 days.

Oxygen is commonly used for the palliation of breathlessness. However, a Cochrane review, which included 35 randomised people with CHF, concluded that there was insufficient evidence for the benefits of oxygen over air for the relief of breathlessness (Cranston, Crockett & Currow 2008). Since then, an adequately powered multi-centre RCT of 239 patients (only 7 with heart disease) has been conducted, comparing oxygen therapy with medical air in palliative patients with breathlessness and a PaO_2 >7.3kPa (normoxaemic/mildly hypoxaemic) (Abernethy *et al.* 2010). Breathlessness improved in both study arms, but neither proved superior to the other. The authors recommend that less burdensome strategies, such as facial airflow from a simple battery-operated hand-held fan, should be considered first. If this is not helpful, then a three-day clinical assessment of the effects of oxygen therapy on the individual patient should be made.

Summary

A community patient with breathlessness and a diagnosis of heart failure requires careful assessment to determine whether the breathlessness is due to the heart failure and, if so, if there is a precipitating cause of the exacerbation. Co-morbid factors need to be identified and appropriately treated. A key aspect of good symptom control of breathlessness due to heart failure is excellent treatment of the heart failure itself. This may include patient education and self-management programmes, lifestyle advice, optimising heart failure medication and, for some patients, cardiac devices and even LVADs or transplants.

Having used all these management strategies, patients are often left with refractory breathlessness. This is a common and chronic problem and it is easy to take a very negative view and think that 'nothing further can be done'. However, there is much that can be done. As with other symptoms, such as pain, investigation should begin with a full holistic assessment (including input from family members and carers), followed by appropriate management of any identified concerns.

Specific recommendations will usually include ensuring that the patient has been on an appropriate cardiac exercise programme, which includes education and psychological support, and ensuring that these messages are reinforced. A simple additional tool is a hand-held fan, which allows them to be in control of their own breathlessness management. Low-dose opioids may be helpful but should be initiated with due caution in patients with renal impairment, which is a common co-morbidity. Oxygen should not be given routinely and, when used, should be started as a trial, with reassessment after three days.

Patients with breathlessness due to chronic heart failure experience considerable distress, often for months or years. Community practitioners have a great deal to offer these patients and their families. Using the tools of good assessment and simple interventions, they can do much to transform these patients' lives.

References

Abernethy, A.P., McDonald, C.F., Frith, P.A., Clark, K., Herndon, J.E., Marcello, J., Young, I.H., Bull, J., Wilcock, A., Booth, S., Wheeler, J.L., Tulsky, J.A., Crockett, A.J. & Currow, D.C. (2010). Effect of palliative oxygen versus room air in relief of breathlessness in patients with refractory dyspnoea: a double-blind, randomised controlled trial. *The Lancet*. **376**, 784–93.

Abernethy, A.P. & Wheeler, J.L. (2008). Total dyspnoea. *Current Opinion in Supportive Palliative Care*. **2**, 110–13.

Bausewein, C., Booth, S., Gysels, M. & Higginson, I. (2008). Non-pharmacological interventions for breathlessness in advanced stages of malignant and non-malignant diseases. *Cochrane Database Systematic Review*. no. 2, p. CD005623

Banerjee, P., Gill, L., Muir, V., Nadar, S., Raja, Y., Goyal, D. & Koganti, S. (2010). Do heart failure patients understand their diagnosis or want to know their prognosis? Heart failure from a patient's perspective. *Clinical Medicine*. **10**, 339–43.

Clark, A.L., Poole-Wilson, P.A. & Coats, A.J. (1996). Exercise limitation in chronic heart failure: central role of the periphery. *Journal of American College of Cardiology*. **28** (5), 1092–102.

Cranston, J.M., Crockett, A. & Currow, D. (2008). Oxygen therapy for dyspnoea in adults. *Cochrane Database of Systematic Reviews*. no. 3, CD004769.

Currow, D., Smith, J., Davidson, P.M., Newton, P., Agar, M.R. & Abernethy, A.P. (2010). Do the trajectories of dyspnea differ in prevalence and intensity by diagnosis at the end of life? A consecutive cohort study. *Journal of Pain and Symptom Management*. **39**, 680–90.

Galbraith, S., Fagan, P., Perkins, P., Lynch, A. & Booth, S. (2010) Does the use of a handheld fan improve chronic dyspnea? A randomized, controlled, crossover trial. *Journal of Pain and Symptom Management*. **39**, 831–38.

George, M. & Linda, H. (2001). Pathophysiology of chronic heart failure. *American Journal of Medicine*. **110** Suppl 7A: 37S–46S.

Goodyer, L.I., Miskelly, F. & Milligan, P. (1995). Does encouraging good compliance improve patients' clinical condition in heart failure? *Br. J. Clin. Pract.* **49**(4), 173–76.

Harrington, D., Anker, S.D. & Coats, A.J. (2001). Preservation of exercise capacity and lack of peripheral changes in asymptomatic patients with severely impaired left ventricular function. *European Heart Journal*. **22**, 392–99.

Jennings, A.L., Davies, A.N., Higgins, J.P., Gibbs, J.S. & Broadley, K.E. (2002). A systematic review of the use of opioids in the management of dyspnoea. *Thorax*. **57**, 939–44.

Jensen, D., Alsuhail, A., Viola, R., Dudgeon, D.J., Webb, K.A. & O'Donnell, D.E. (2012). Inhaled fentanyl citrate improves exercise endurance during high-intensity, constant work-rate cycle exercise in COPD. *Journal of Pain and Symptom Management*. **3**(4), 706–19.

Johnson, M.J., McDonagh, T.A., Harkness, A., McKay, S.E. & Dargie, H.J. (2002). Morphine for the relief of breathlessness in patients with chronic heart failure – a pilot study, *European Journal of Heart Failure*. **4**, 753–56.

National Institute for Health and Clinical Excellence (NICE) (2010) Management of Chronic Heart Failure in Adults in Primary and Secondary Care. NICE Clinical Guideline 108.

New York Heart Association (1994). *Nomenclature and Criteria for Diagnosis of Diseases of the Heart and Great Vessels*, 9th ed. Boston, MA: Little, Brown.

Oxberry, S.G., Torgerson, D.J., Bland, J.M., Clark, A.L., Cleland, J.G. & Johnson, M.J. (2011). Short-term opioids for breathlessness in stable chronic heart failure: a randomized controlled trial. *European Journal of Heart Failure*. **13**, 1006–12.

Oxberry, S.G., Bland, J.M., Clark, A.L., Cleland, J.G. & Johnson, M.J. (2013) Repeat dose opioids may be effective for breathlessness in chronic heart failure if given for long enough. *Journal of Palliative Medicine*. **16** (3), 250–55.

Packer, M. (1992). The neurohormonal hypothesis: a theory to explain the mechanism of disease progression in heart failure. *Journal of American College of Cardiology*. **20** (1), 248–54.

Pitsis, A.A. (2008). Heart and lung transplantation: new flavours from old recipes. *Hellenic Journal of Cardiology*. **49**, 238–40.

Rees, K., Taylor, R.R.S., Singh, S., Coats, A.J. & Ebrahim, S. (2009). Exercise based rehabilitation for heart failure (Review), *Cochrane Database of Systematic Reviews* no. 3, p. CD003331.

Reviriego, M. (2011). A review of recommendations for cardiac resynchronisation therapy in patients with atrial fibrilation. *E-Journal of Cardiology Practice*. **9** (36).

Sullivan, M.J., Wood, L., Terry, J., Brantley, J., Charles, A., McGee, V., Johnson, D., Krucoff, M.W., Rosenberg, B., Bosworth, H.B., Adams, K. & Cuffe, M. S. (2009). The Support, Education, and Research in Chronic Heart Failure Study (SEARCH): a mindfulness-based psychoeducational intervention improves depression and clinical symptoms in patients with chronic heart failure. *American Heart* **157**, 84–90.

Yu, D.S., Lee, D.T., Woo, J. & Hui, E. (2007). Non-pharmacological interventions in older people with heart failure: effects of exercise training and relaxation therapy. *Gerontology*. **53**, 74–81.

6

Breathlessness and interstitial lung disease

Annette Duck

Patient perspective: Living with idiopathic pulmonary fibrosis

My life was so different before the onset of idiopathic pulmonary fibrosis (IPF). Having retired in 1999 at the age of 61, I was healthy and energetic. To maintain these conditions, my wife and I set our sights on 'doing what we can whilst we can'. Living close to the Peak District, we enjoyed a fair amount of walking. It was on one such walk that for the very first time I experienced breathlessness whilst climbing a relatively gently sloping footpath. It did not register at the time that something might be wrong and we continued with our normal lifestyle.

In the early part of 2004, I was in hospital for a painful right calf and a nurse noticed that my breathing was laboured, although I was not aware of this. A chest x-ray revealed shadows on both lungs and I was referred to the hospital's chest clinic, where my condition was diagnosed as IPF. I attended the clinic for the next three years and had regular lung function tests but little else. The prescribed treatment was the use of inhalers. However, I was concerned that this was achieving very little; I was still experiencing shortness of breath on little exertion. I was transferred to a specialist lung centre and almost immediately my medication was changed to include steroids, aziathioprine and various other drugs.

The impact of breathlessness

Between 2004 and 2008, my breathlessness was having a greater effect on my life. Activities that had previously not been a problem were causing me considerable discomfort, and much of my fitness programme at the gym was being reduced or dropped completely. Gradually my condition has worsened considerably and even mild effort now causes severe breathlessness. Getting showered and dressed, getting into the car, going to the shops and so on necessitate using my oxygen supply at the highest level of 8 litres per minute, and even then I need to rest at regular intervals.

My days begin with a shower and getting dressed. Both activities cause me to be breathless. However, in the case of showering, I have seen a remarkable improvement by using a lightweight, purpose-made shower stool that enables me to sit down in the shower. A further benefit comes from using my oxygen whilst showering. I continue with the oxygen whilst getting dressed and my wife simplifies the process by arranging my clothes so that I do not need to access drawers and wardrobes.

In overall terms I attempt to avoid severe episodes of breathlessness by resting at regular intervals, always using my oxygen at the recommended levels and by using lifts rather than staircases. I plan ahead for events away from home and make use of any mobility aids supplied by event organisers and large shops. I rarely suffer anxiety arising from IPF but when I do so, I sit down, and inhale deeply via my nostrils and exhale via my mouth.

Needing oxygen at home

In April 2008, I took an Oxygen Assessment Test and as a result I was prescribed Home and Ambulatory Oxygen for 16 hours per day at a rate of 1 litre per minute at rest and 6 litres per minute for exercise. This has recently been increased to 2 litres per minute and 8 litres per minute, respectively.

At home I have two supplies of oxygen. One is via a concentrator, which I rely on whilst asleep and during the day whilst in the house. My second supply is in liquid oxygen form, and this is ambulatory oxygen for use whilst engaged in any form of activity away from home. Without oxygen, much of my mobility would not be possible.

Keeping active and staying positive

On the upside I remain very positive, I love the company of people, enjoy holidays and derive a lot of support from the staff at the specialist lung centre. I do not dwell on my problem but I do miss not being able to work alongside my wife and I know that my daughter worries about me. I have found from experience and discussion with other IPF patients that there are many ways in which to improve my mobility and attitude towards the disease. Most important in dealing with IPF is a positive 'can do' approach, which enables me to have control of the condition and which empowers me to continue with my life as normally as possible.

Breathlessness in interstitial lung disease

Introduction

Interstitial lung disease (ILD) is the umbrella term given to a collection of restrictive lung disorders that result in scarring of the lung parenchyma. The physiological disease processes also include the local blood circulatory system and interstitial space between the alveoli and capillary circulation. This ultimately interferes with oxygen diffusion into the blood circulation. It also leads to reduced compliance and elasticity of the lung, resulting in breathlessness.

Epidemiology

Over 200 different types of ILDs have been reported in the medical literature and this can cause confusion in diagnosis and treatment management. Most types are quite rare and most general clinicians will come into contact with only the most common ones. Broadly speaking, ILD can be categorised into the idiopathic interstitial pneumonias (IIPs) and the others, which include conditions such as sarcoidosis, connective tissue related disorders, occupational or environmentally induced ILD (linked to activities such as woodworking or metalworking), and hypersensitivity pneumonitis (HP), also known as pigeon fancier's or farmer's lung (ATS 2000). Many of the ILDs include the IIPs, of which more than half are estimated to include idiopathic pulmonary fibrosis (IPF). IPF is the most common form of ILD and the one that most clinicians will come across in practice.

In the past, IPF has also been known as pulmonary fibrosis and cryptogenic fibrosing alveolitis (CFA), but since the reclassification of the ILDs (ATS 2000), it has been labelled as IPF. Other ILDs that carry a similar symptom burden include conditions known as non-specific interstitial pneumonitis (NSIP), acute interstitial pneumonitis (AIP), hypersensitivity pneumonitis (HP) and others.

A detailed account of the classification of the ILDs is not the purpose of this chapter. IPF is the most common form of ILD, although other ILDs have similar symptoms of breathlessness and psychological impact in the advanced stages of disease.

IPF starts insidiously, in the 50–80 age group, and there are currently no good treatments, meaning that it is incurable. The cause of IPF remains unknown. It is not specific to smokers, as it can also affect lifelong non-smokers. One study (Raghu *et al.* 2006) estimated the prevalence between 14.0 and 42.7 per 100,000 in the USA. Meanwhile, a British study (Gribben *et al.* 2006) estimated that the incidence of IPF increased by 11% from 1991 and 2003, showing that this disease is either on the increase or is becoming better diagnosed.

Currently, 1500 people living in the UK have a diagnosis of IPF, with more than 5000 new cases diagnosed each year (Navaratnam *et al.* 2011). The current median life expectancy of three years means that 5000 people will die each year from IPF. More people will die from IPF clinical syndrome than from ovarian cancer, lymphoma, leukaemia, mesothelioma or kidney cancer. The incidence of IPF increased in primary care six-fold between 1968 and 2008, and rose by 35% from 2000 to 2008 (Navaratnam *et al.* 2011). These statistics highlight the importance of clinicians gaining an understanding of the disease, as they will need to monitor and manage terminally ill patients with IPF.

Pathophysiology of ILD and IPF

In all ILDs the structure of the lung is altered and this contributes to breathlessness. Although the specific cause of IPF remains unknown, there are several hypotheses that explain the mechanism of disease. We know that scarring occurs in the lung following an injury or insult, and this is thought to be related to an altered phenotype in the alveolar epithelium (Hoo & Whtye 2011). It is not known whether this could be one insult or a repetitive injury. The abnormal repair, along with suppressed fibrinolytic activity resulting in fibrin deposition in the interstitium and alveoli, may be related to the development of IPF (Chapman, Allen & Stone 1986).

Another hypothesis is that oxidative imbalances in the lower airways have an effect on TGFβ, which can affect pulmonary cell growth factors, creating an environment that encourages fibrin growth (Demedts *et al.*

2005). Demedts and colleagues demonstrated the positive effects of using the anti-oxidant drug N-acetylcysteine, which is now being re-tested in the PANTHER study in the USA. Bacterial colonisation in the lower airways has been associated with higher levels of an anti-inflammatory cytokine called interleukin 1, with 36% of IPF patients having positive bacterial cultures that might be driving the disease (Richter, Stockley & Harper 2009). It is unclear whether these higher bacterial levels are a cause of IPF or an incidental finding in damaged lung parenchyma. As yet the cause of IPF remains elusive, and the search for curative treatment therefore continues. For this reason, management of patients with IPF is currently based on strategies that support the patient and relieve breathlessness. The mechanisms involved in other ILDs are slightly different. For instance, in sarcoidosis normal lung tissue is replaced by characteristic granulomas, thus reducing the amount of normal tissue available for respiration. In connective tissue-related disease, the systemic peripheral capillary circulation is affected throughout the body including the lung.

Mechanisms of breathlessness in ILD

In most ILDs, breathlessness is thought to be mainly caused by a combination of hypoxia and reduced compliance of lung tissue. Fibrosis and scarring leads to a thickened membrane at the alveolar capillary junction, resulting in reduced diffusion of oxygen into the blood circulation. Exercise-induced breathlessness may be the first symptom experienced by patients with ILD, as the muscles' oxygen demand is increased during exercise. If left untreated, the scarring process will continue, causing breathlessness on minimal exertion and finally at rest. Scarring also results in reduced compliance or increased 'stiffness' of the lung tissue, making the work of breathing harder because the lungs are not as easily inflated during inspiration. With progressive scarring and decreased lung compliance, resistance increases in the pulmonary circulation. This raises pressure in the cardio-pulmonary circulation, eventually leading to pulmonary hypertension, which is thought to be a contributing factor in breathlessness in advanced disease. A combination of all these mechanisms means that the patient tends to experience extreme breathlessness on exercise and when completing the routine activities of daily living. Cough can also be a troublesome symptom in IPF.

Reflection point

Some patients with ILD experience breathlessness without significant hypoxia. These patients usually have no history of smoking, and their breathlessness is associated with the small airways becoming stiff as the disease advances. This stiffness makes inspiration difficult, so the patient takes rapid inspiratory breaths and may speak using short sentences with intermittent coughing.

Assessment of ILD in the community

Many patients with ILD, who initially present with breathlessness on exertion in primary care, are misdiagnosed (Schoenheit, Becattelli & Cohen 2011). They may make several visits to their GP before being diagnosed, which may occur following an acute event that requires hospitalisation. Many are smokers or ex-smokers and may therefore be treated with inappropriate inhaler therapies that delay appropriate assessment, diagnosis and treatment.

An ILD diagnosis can only be made on radiology and performance of transfer factor on lung function. Spirometry (usually performed in general practice) may be normal in mild to moderate ILD. A patient describing breathlessness on exertion, who may or may not have a cough, should therefore be referred for a routine chest X-ray. Anything other than a normal chest X-ray from a patient describing breathlessness should be referred to a chest physician for investigation with a high-resolution chest tomography (HRCT) scan, which will confirm a diagnosis. A holistic assessment of the patient presenting in primary care is essential. As explained earlier, breathlessness is a common symptom in COPD, heart failure and other terminal diseases and as such should be intensely investigated to find the definitive cause. As ILD and in particular IPF can occur in the older population, it may occur in conjunction with COPD or heart failure, and the degree of breathlessness associated with each disease can only be ascertained by means of careful assessment.

Pharmaceutical management of ILD

Many ILDs are treatable if diagnosed early, so it is important that these diseases are detected and treated before severe scarring has occurred. Guideline recommended treatments are available for sarcoidosis, connective tissue related ILDs, NSIP, HP and IPF (BTS 2008; NICE 2013). Sarcoidosis usually presents in the younger population and mostly responds to therapy. Due to the high rate of spontaneous remission, sarcoidosis is only treated if there are significant symptoms or progressive disease. Often all that is required is a course of steroids, with monitoring by radiology and lung function. Occasionally it is necessary to use an additional therapy such as methotrexate, which needs careful blood monitoring for cellular counts and patient tolerance.

HP, which used to be known as extrinsic allergic alveolitis (EAA) or pigeon fancier's or farmer's lung, usually responds to removal of the offending antigen and a course of steroids, depending upon response to therapy. The offending antigen is not always identified so it is essential to take a careful history of the working environment and leisure pursuits in order to advise, monitor and manage these patients. Occasionally it is difficult to stabilise the disease without using multiple therapies, and very occasionally lung transplantation will need to be considered.

NSIP is similar in symptom presentation and radiology, offering only subtle differences on HRCT that can usually be discerned only by an experienced radiologist. It has therefore been suggested by Flaherty *et al.* (2004) that all patients suspected of having an ILD should be referred to a specialist multidisciplinary team, which includes a specialist radiologist and pathologist, for diagnosis. Unlike IPF, NSIP responds to therapy and is treated with steroids and a combination of immuno-suppressive therapy, usually azathioprine (BTS 2008). It is vital to carefully monitor the patient's response to the side-effects of each therapy. These include diabetes, hypertension, cataracts, osteoporosis and weight gain with prednisolone, and pan-cytopenia, liver function abnormalities and myalagia with azathioprine (BTS 2008).

The most recent IPF publication (ATS/ERS/JRS/ALAT 2011) guideline recommends that all patients diagnosed with IPF should be offered the opportunity to enter a clinical trial. However, this is not feasible for many patients with IPF, given the difficulties of late diagnosis, meeting the inclusion/exclusion criteria of the trials and travelling to the trial study centres. Many patients with IPF are still being treated with triple therapy, which includes prednisolone, azathioprine and N-acetylcysteine (NAC). The triple therapy arm was recently stopped by the data monitoring committee in the PANTHER study, due to an increased number of deaths in this arm of the study. Meanwhile, the NAC versus placebo arm was allowed to continue. This result has led to the British Thoracic Society's additional 2011 recommendation that no newly diagnosed IPF patients should be started on triple therapy, and those already on these drugs should be made aware of the British Thoracic Society's post-PANTHER 2011 recommendations. In the light of the patient's exacerbation history, the patient and physician should make a joint decision about whether or not the patient should stay on this treatment.

A new drug called pirfenidone has recently been licensed by NICE for use in IPF (NICE 2013). In clinical trials, this anti-fibrotic drug with anti-inflammatory properties has been found to slow down the rate of decline in forced vital capacity (FVC), promising hope for the development of a new range of drugs for the treatment of IPF.

Lung transplantation offers a chance of a longer-term survival and any patient diagnosed with IPF, without any other absolute contra-indications (discuss with local transplant centre), should be considered for a lung transplant (Glanville & Estenne 2003; NICE 2013). All patients diagnosed with IPF and advanced ILD should be offered best supportive care (BTS 2008), including breathlessness and cough management and palliative care.

Pharmacological management of breathlessness

Oxygen therapy

Central to managing breathlessness in all ILDs is ensuring that oxygen therapy is appropriate for the stage of the disease. Exercise-induced hypoxia is the hallmark of this lung disease. It is therefore mandatory for careful regular oxygen assessments to be conducted while patients are exercising. Oxygen saturations at rest may be normal, and will not indicate the degree of breathlessness experienced while performing the normal activities of daily living. Ideally, formal ambulatory oxygen assessments should be carried out at a local oxygen assessment centre. Checking oxygen saturations with pulse oximetry while a patient is walking up the stairs or around the home will demonstrate whether or not they are experiencing exercise-induced hypoxia.

During exercise or exertion, patients' oxygen saturation may deteriorate from being within normal limits to SpO_2 levels between 60 and 70. These patients will need ambulatory oxygen to walk outside their homes and to perform most activities of daily living (Frank *et al.* 2012). They will also need regular (often three-monthly) ambulatory oxygen review to prevent extreme exercise-induced hypoxia, which may cause panic and result in emergency hospital admission.

In advanced disease, ILD patients will also need oxygen therapy at rest and should be assessed for long-term oxygen therapy (LTOT) as per British Thoracic Society (2006) guidelines, similarly to patients with COPD. Patients with ILD may require two different oxygen prescriptions – one for resting, sitting and sleeping, and one for ambulatory use and completing activities of daily living in the home. In the terminal phase, patients often prefer oxygen delivered under pressure. They may therefore switch from high-flow nasal cannula to a venturi mask that will deliver a higher total gas flow, thus aiding inspiration against fibrotic stiff lungs. High-flow oxygen delivered through a high-flow oxygen-generating machine can reduce the symptoms of breathlessness but is not sustainable outside hospital. It signals terminal disease and the need to commence pharmacological management strategies, usually through a syringe driver.

Reflection point Reflection point Reflection point

Focus of breathlessness, hypoxia and oxygen therapy

It is important to assess all patients with IPF and breathlessness on exertion for exercise-induced hypoxia. Patients are likely to experience exercise-induced hypoxia that can significantly reduce their exercise ability. They should be assessed with either a shuttle walk or six-minute walk test to evaluate whether they are experiencing breathlessness associated with hypoxia.

- A shuttle walk test is an exercise assessment test. The patient is instructed to walk at a predetermined pace, which increases with distance and time. Oxygen levels are monitored by pulse oximetry as patients are challenged to exercise to their limits.
- A six-minute walk test with pulse oximetry is a self-paced walk test and is useful for titrating ambulatory oxygen.

It is important to explain to the patient that, although ambulatory oxygen may not stop oxygen desaturation on exercise, it will raise the baseline oxygen level, maintain higher capillary oxygen levels for longer and enable a faster recovery rate, thus improving exercise performance overall.

The evidence for pharmacological management

The evidence for pharmacological management of breathlessness in ILD is sparse, and most pharmacological management strategies used in clinical practice have been extrapolated from the evidence in COPD and lung cancer. Breathlessness is perceived in the respiratory centre in the brainstem, which is rich in opioid receptors, and this may explain why opioids can reduce the sensation of breathlessness. The lungs also contain some opioid receptors and it has been demonstrated in a systematic review (Jennings *et al.* 2002) that morphine is useful in reducing the sensation of exercise-induced breathlessness, although the review also demonstrated that more evidence was needed to substantiate the existing evidence. Unfortunately the studies using nebulised morphine were not so convincing. Bruera *et al.* (1993) showed that patients with resting breathlessness, who were already using morphine for pain, experienced a reduction in breathlessness with a 50% increase in morphine, with no decrease in oxygen saturation and no increase in respiratory depression

Palliation of breathlessness in ILD with pharmacological preparations should be offered to patients if breathlessness is not controlled by oxygen. The maximum amount of oxygen that can currently be administered in the community is 16 litres/min issued by two high-flow concentrators. This is sufficient to drive a 60% venturi mask. Using a non-rebreathe mask with a portable cylinder or liquid oxygen is useful for moving around the home, as it can deliver between 80 and 90% oxygen at 15 litres/min. Before patients are using this amount of oxygen they need to start using pharmacological preparations to control breathlessness. Morphine (in the form of oramorph) should be offered to patients and increased if needed to blunt the sensation of breathlessness. The evidence for using benzodiazepines to reduce breathlessness in advancing disease is not strong, but they should be considered for patients experiencing panic and anxiety associated with breathlessness. Sublingual lorazepam can help reduce anxiety associated with breathlessness. In terminal disease, extreme breathlessness should be managed (as in any other terminal illness) with a diamorphine and midazolam infusion pump.

Non-pharmacological management of breathlessness

Non-pharmacological management of breathlessness in ILDs is similar to that used in any other condition causing breathlessness (see Chapter 8). For those with late stage disease and disabling breathlessness, pacing and prioritising activities, so as not to cause undue lethargy and exhaustion, is the first consideration. Not having too high an expectation of what can be achieved is fundamental to maintaining a positive attitude despite having breathlessness. Individuals develop different coping strategies according to their personality. However, suggestions from a supportive healthcare practitioner are likely to help any patient who has to adjust to debilitating breathlessness. Doing things slowly, stopping and resting, and avoiding the need to rush are all techniques that need to be mastered to enable patients to complete their chosen activities (see Chapter 8 for energy conservation techniques). Patients need to feel 'in control' if they are to adjust, and they can only be 'in control' if they learn to do things despite being breathless.

Opening windows to encourage movement of room air and the use of fans (Bruera *et al.* 1993) have been described as helpful. Participation in an ILD support group or pulmonary rehabilitation programme may also be helpful, as patients can learn from healthcare practitioners and other patients how to continue to do the things that are important to them. An evidence base for the value of patients with ILD attending pulmonary rehabilitation is developing and early results are promising (Nishiyama *et al.* 2000). Participation in a pulmonary rehabilitation programme may therefore be helpful for some patients. Pulmonary rehabilitation will have benefits for exercise tolerance if completed early in the disease trajectory; for those patients referred later in their disease progression, pulmonary rehabilitation may simply be a useful way to learn the non-pharmacological techniques to manage breathlessness and the ensuing debility. For these reasons, it is advisable to refer patients early in the course of their disease and pulmonary rehabilitation programmes would do well to fast-track IPF patients for maximum benefit.

Management of IPF exacerbations

It is now thought that patients with IPF develop exacerbations similar to those experienced with COPD. Patients undoubtedly experience periods of sudden increased breathlessness, often with no apparent infection, when their oxygen demand suddenly increases. During these episodes, patients initially present in primary care and should be assessed not only for infection but also for a pulmonary embolism, which is not uncommon in patients with IPF (Nathan *et al.* 2003). Any signs of infection, including increased production of discoloured phlegm, tachypnoea, pyrexia, increased inflammatory markers or raised white cell count, need prompt antibiotic therapy. Unlike patients with COPD, patients with IPF do not recover to a pre-exacerbation state, but remain on a reduced level of functional ability. If infection and pulmonary embolism are successfully treated or ruled out, the patient may spontaneously stabilise on a lower level of function. Alternatively, they may continue on a rapid spiral of decline, often unresponsive to the cortico-steroids used as an attempt at rescue therapy. The course of IPF is unpredictable and varies from patient to patient.

Reflection point Reflection point Reflection point

Consider how an exacerbation might present in a patient with ILD and in a patient with COPD. What might some of the similarities and differences be?

Summary

Diagnosing, assessing, monitoring and managing patients with ILDs can be confusing but rewarding. It is not necessary to understand the complexities of the different ILD diagnoses in order to support and manage a breathless patient with ILD. However, it is vital to understand the importance of getting a firm diagnosis, as many ILDs respond to appropriate treatment. Once a diagnosis has been made and appropriate treatment has been instigated, the principles of breathlessness assessment are similar for most ILDs. In order to manage the condition effectively, it is crucial to determine whether the breathlessness is due to deteriorating disease or another superimposed cause (such as infection or pulmonary embolism) or other co-morbidities (such as co-existing heart failure or COPD). When in doubt, it is always appropriate to refer on to specialist teams.

References

American Thoracic Society (ATS). (2000). Idiopathic Pulmonary Fibrosis: Diagnosis and treatment international consensus statement. *American Journal of Critical Care Medicine*. **161**, 646–64.

American Thoracic Society (ATS)/European Respiratory Society (ERS)/Japanese Respiratory Society (JRS)/Latin American Thoracic Society (ALAT). (2011). Statement: Idiopathic pulmonary fibrosis: Evidence-based guidelines for diagnosis and management. *American Journal of Critical Care Medicine*. **183**, 788–824.

British Thoracic Society (BTS). (2006). Clinical Component for the Home Oxygen Service in England and Wales. Downloaded from http://www.brit-thoracic.org.uk/Portals/0/Clinical%20Information/Home%20Oxygen%20Service/clinical%20adultoxygenjan06.pdf. 22/01/12.

British Thoracic Society (BTS). (2008). Interstitial lung disease guideline: the British Thoracic Society in collaboration with the Thoracic Society of Australia, and New Zealand and the Irish Thoracic Society. *Thorax*. **63**, v1–v58.

Bruera, E., MacEachern, T., Ripamonti, C. & Hanson, J. (1993). Subcutaneous morphine for dyspnoea in cancer patients. *Annals of Oncology*. **119**, 906–7.

Chapman, H., Allen, C. & Stone, O. (1986). Abnormalities in pathways of alveolar fibrin turnover among patients with interstitial lung disease. *American Review of Respiratory Disease*. **133**, 437–43.

Demedts, M., Behr, J., Buhl, R., Costabel, U., Dekhuijzen, R., Jansen, H., MacNee, W., Thomeer, M., Walleart, B. & Laurent, F. (2005). High-dose acetylcysteine in idiopathic pulmonary fibrosis. *New England Journal of Medicine*. **353**, 2229–42.

Flaherty K.R., King T.E. Jr & Raghu, G. (2004). Idiopathic interstitial pneumonia: what is the effect of a multidisciplinary approach to diagnosis? *American Journal of Respiratory Critical Care Medicine*. **170**, 904–10.

Frank, R.C., Hicks, S., Duck, A.M., Spencer, L., Leonard, C.T. & Barnett, E. (2021). Ambulatory oxygen in IPF: of what benefit? *European Respiratory Journal*. **40** (1), 269–70.

Glanville, A. & Estenne, M. (2003). Indications, patient selection and timing of referral for lung transplantation. *European Respiratory Journal*. **22**, 845–52.

Gribbon, J., Hubbard, R., Lo Jouno, I., Smith, C., West, J. & Tata, L. (2006). Incidence and mortality of idiopathic pulmonary fibrosis and sarcoidosis in the UK. *Thorax*. **61**, 980–85.

Hoo, Z. & Whyte, M. (2011). Idiopathic pulmonary fibrosis. *Thorax* doi: 10.1136. Downloaded from BMJ Com. 22/01/2012.

Jennings, A., Davies, A., Higgins, J., Gibbs, J. & Broadley, K. (2002). A systematic review of the use of opioids in the management of dyspnoea. *Thorax*. **57** (11), 939–44.

Nathan S., Barnett, S., Urban, B., Nowalk, C., Moran, B. & Burton, N. (2003). Pulmonary embolism in idiopathic pulmonary fibrosis lung transplant recipients. *Chest*. **123**,1758–63.

Navaratnam, V., Fleming, K. & West, J. (2011). The rising incidence of idiopathic pulmonary fibrosis in the UK. *Thorax*. **66**, 462–67.

NICE (2013) Idiopathic pulmonary fibrosis: the diagnosis and management of suspected idiopathic pulmonary fibrosis, clinical guidelines. CG163. June.

Nishiyama, O., Kondoh, Y., Kimura, T., Kato, K., Kataoka, K., Ogawa, T., Watanbe, F., Arizono, S., Nishurma, K. & Taniguchi, H. (2008). Effects of pulmonary rehabilitation in patients with idiopathic pulmonary fibrosis. *Respirology*, **13**, 394–9.

Raghu, G., Weycker, D., Edelsberg, J., Bradford, W. & Oster, G. (2006). Incidence and prevalence of idiopathic pulmonary fibrosis. *American Journal of Respiratory and Critical Care Medicine*. **174**, 810–16.

Richter, A., Stockley, R. & Harper, L. (2009). Pulmonary infection in Wegener Granulomatosis and idiopathic pulmonary fibrosis. *Thorax*. **64**, 692–97.

Schoenheit, G., Becattelli, I. & Cohen, A. (2011). Living with idiopathic pulmonary fibrosis: an in-depth qualitative survey of European patients. *Chronic Respiratory Disease*. **8** (4), 225–31.

7

Breathlessness and pulmonary hypertension

Iain Armstrong

Patient perspective: Living with pulmonary hypertension

Growing up, studying and working

When I was three or four years old, I was walking and trying to keep up with others when it was noticed that I got breathless a lot, turned purple/blue and would sometimes even sit down and refuse to get up for a while. I was taken to a local doctor who referred me to a hospital where they later carried out a series of observations (catheter into heart via arm/groin) and discovered that I had a hole in my heart (otherwise known as a ventricular septal defect or VSD) and had developed Eisenmenger's.

I found my first stay in this London hospital in the early 1960s daunting. I felt deserted, as my mother was not allowed to stay with me. I still remember the clanging sound that the medical injection trolley made as it came up the ward. It would cause me to panic the nearer it got, as I feared it was time for another injection. Later, my fear of injections would cause me to worry for days before an annual check-up. It was many years afterwards that a doctor taught me distraction techniques to get over having injections. It was great to get over this phobia and now I don't worry before getting an injection.

When I was about 12 years old, I got the first signs of an aspect of my condition that I would have to learn to cope with for the rest of my life. While having a bath, I coughed up blood. Although at first I was shocked and confused, I kept it to myself, as I did not wish to upset my parents. Fortunately the bleeding stopped soon afterwards.

When I was preparing for my university finals, the bleeding from the lung (haemoptysis) became more of a problem. I went to see the university doctor who thought I had swallowed a chicken bone after eating a curry the previous night and thought it would quickly heal. However, during my last two or three exams the bleeding was still a problem so I had to just swallow the blood and try to calm down (which was very difficult in an exam).

After university, I quickly found out that it was difficult to get a job with any large commercial company, as I tended to get rejected as soon as they found out about my heart condition. So I ended up either working for the NHS or self-employed, doing contracting work. Nearly all my jobs came through recommendations. I am glad that there are anti-discriminatory laws in place now to help stop this kind of prejudiced behaviour towards disabled people.

At times, the haemoptysis got so bad that it was very difficult to control. I mostly had to lie very still and calm, and learn to control my breathing so that it was very slow and steady. It was important not to cough, as this could set off an episode of heavy bleeding. Suppressing coughing was very difficult, as my throat was burning due to the irritating effects of the blood. It required grim determination to ignore this sensation. If the haemoptysis got out of control I would sometimes end up dosed with morphine in a high dependency unit.

General aspects of living with VSD, Eisenmenger's and pulmonary hypertension

From a very early age, I remember getting out of breath if I ran for any length of time, or walked up a steep slope or at speed. I would also get breathless if I climbed more than one flight of stairs. As I got older, these symptoms got worse and I would have to do less and less to get breathless and tired out. Now I find that if I exert myself one day, then I will need to rest the next day or so to recover. Nowadays, I have to take one or more rests if I wash up or do other such tasks.

In my later life when haemoptysis was more of an issue, I had to learn to monitor my level of exertion so I could avoid initiating further episodes. I learned to sense the pressure in my lungs and to some extent control my heart rate. I could feel the pressure rising internally as a feeling of pushing against what I suspected was old scar tissue in my lungs. If I sensed this, I would try to calm down and I could often avoid a major attack. I would mainly miss the signs if I had become angry or had been over-exerting myself and was distracted. Sometimes I would wake in the night with the oh-so-familiar panic-filled sensation of a miniature aerosol going off in my lungs. I would have to calm myself as quickly as possible and take stock, and then wait and see if I could cope or whether we would have to phone for an ambulance.

One of the hardest things to cope with was the uncertainty of this condition. I was unsure on a daily basis if I was going to have an episode of haemoptysis, as it could occur at any time and I always had to be on the lookout for it. Sometimes worries about whether I would wake up the next day also preyed on my mind. In the end I learned to some extent to just bury and suppress these feelings and get on with life.

Diagnosing pulmonary hypertension

Pulmonary hypertension (PH) is a serious, life-limiting condition that is often diagnosed long after symptoms first occur. Studies have estimated that the average time from first visiting a doctor to diagnosis is between 2 and 2.5 years (Humbert *et al.* 2006, PHA UK 2010). The non-specific symptoms of PH mean that it is often initially misdiagnosed as a respiratory condition such as asthma or chronic obstructive pulmonary disease (COPD), or a heart condition such as angina. The symptoms of PH include breathlessness, syncope, chest pain and tightness, and fatigue (McGoon *et al.* 2004).

PH is characterised by pulmonary vascular remodelling leading to increasing pulmonary vascular resistance, and ultimately right heart failure. The main pathophysiological characteristics of PH are the narrowing and thickening of the pulmonary artery walls. These changes are caused by a number of factors, including pulmonary vasoconstriction, hypertrophy and fibrosis.

Diagnosis of PH involves confirming the disease, determining the underlying aetiology (clinical classification) and evaluating the severity of the disease (McGoon *et al.* 2004). PH is a heterogeneous condition that is classified into different groups. The classification of PH requires an accurate patient history, careful examination and interpretation of a variety of investigations. Table 7.1 (on page 103) describes the different groups in the clinical classification of PH.

A number of pathophysiological factors are involved in the genesis of PH.

Firstly, pulmonary vasoconstriction results in a narrowing of the pulmonary arterioles. Hypertrophy refers to enlargement of the cells in the pulmonary artery wall. Fibrosis is the development of excess fibrous tissue in the pulmonary artery wall. Inflammation and thrombosis also contribute to the narrowing and thickening of the pulmonary arterial wall. This thickening of the arterial wall is known as vascular remodelling. It remains uncertain what triggers the remodelling of the pulmonary arterial wall in PH. It can occur in response to injury to the arterial wall or to certain stimuli, such as hypoxia.

In PH, progressive changes to the pulmonary vasculature occur as a response to increased blood pressure in the pulmonary arteries. The vessel wall becomes thicker in order to withstand greater pressure within the arterial lumen, which in turn leads to greater pulmonary vascular resistance. Eventually, increased pulmonary vascular resistance leads to right heart failure.

Pulmonary hypertension is defined as a mean pulmonary artery pressure (MPAP) ≥25mmHg at rest or 30mmHg on exercise (Humbert *et al.* 2006). The World Health Organisation (WHO) recently reclassified pulmonary hypertension and identified five major groups (see Table 7.1). This classification illustrates the importance of identifying the cause of PH when defining treatment. Patients with chronic thromboembolic pulmonary hypertension (CTEPH) can potentially be cured by surgery. PH is a challenging disease to diagnose, accurately classify and treat.

The diagnostic process currently requires invasive investigations, and the treatments are effective but often complex. Until the advent of transplantation in the 1980s, there was no specific treatment for PH. The last two decades have seen the development of new therapies that have been shown to improve the symptoms and survival of patients with PH. Patients with severe disease have a five-year survival rate of only 27% with supportive treatment, but this increases to 54% with certain targeted therapies (McGoon *et al.* 2009). These treatments require significant expertise. For this reason, investigation and treatment of certain forms of PH are currently focused at nationally designated specialist centres. In the UK, centres currently exist in London, Cambridge, Sheffield, Newcastle and Glasgow. There is also a specialist centre in Dublin, Ireland.

Table 7.1: Clinical classifications of PH
(Adapted from Simonneau *et al.* 2009)

Group	Clinical classification
I	Pulmonary arterial hypertension
I' *	Pulmonary veno-occlusive disease and/or pulmonary capillary haemangiomatosis – both very rare
II	Pulmonary hypertension due to left heart disease
III	Pulmonary hypertension due to lung disease and/or hypoxia
IV	Chronic thromboembolic pulmonary hypertension
V	PH with unclear or multifactorial mechanisms

** Group I' is a sub-group of Group I. PVOD and PCH are both extremely rare.*

Approach to diagnosing PH

It is important to diagnose PH at an early stage, as advanced disease is linked to a poorer prognosis (McLaughlin *et al.* 2009). Early diagnosis depends on systematically evaluating patients who are breathless and screening patients who are at increased risk of developing PH. A number of conditions such as connective tissue disease (particularly systemic sclerosis), previous pulmonary embolism and portal hypertension (seen in patients with chronic liver disease) are associated with an increased risk of developing forms of pre-capillary PH for which specific therapies are available (Galiè *et al.* 2009). Identifying patients with PH and then accurately identifying the underlying cause of their PH is the key to managing the condition successfully. PH should be considered in all patients with unexplained progressive breathlessness. When the cause of PH is unknown and other conditions have been ruled out, idiopathic pulmonary arterial hypertension (IPAH) is diagnosed.

Route to diagnosis

There are usually three ways in which patients with suspected PH are identified:

1. Patient presents with typical symptoms of PH, such as progressive breathlessness
2. Screening identifies suspected PH
3. Suspected PH is found during an unrelated investigation.

Patients may present with unexplained breathlessness on exertion that has typically progressed over a number of months or even years. There may also be symptoms such as fatigue, exertional chest pain and syncope. Patients may initially be treated for common causes of breathlessness, such as asthma or COPD. However, patients with pre-capillary PH will not respond to these treatments and their symptoms will progress. Diagnosis is then usually made following referral for specialist evaluation. Patients will then undergo a number of systematic tests, including a variety of imaging investigations as well as right heart catheterisation (the 'gold standard' test for confirming a PH diagnosis).

At-risk individuals (for example, those with connective tissue diseases associated with PH such as systemic sclerosis) should be regularly screened for PH. If screening investigations suggest the possibility of PH, this may need to be confirmed with right heart catheterisation (RHC).

Investigative tests

There are a number of investigations that aim to confirm a diagnosis of PH, and determine the underlying aetiology of the condition and the severity of the disease. Investigations to confirm the diagnosis and identify the cause of PH include:

- Blood tests
- Electrocardiogram (ECG)
- Echocardiogram
- Pulmonary function tests
- Exercise tests
- Chest X-ray
- CT scan
- MRI scan
- Ventilation–perfusion scan
- Pulmonary angiography
- Right heart catheterisation.

Each patient may have slightly different investigations, depending on their underlying conditions and the suspected type of PH. However, it is essential that all patients are systematically evaluated and that the results of the investigations are interpreted by specialist clinicians who are experienced in managing patients with PH.

The most important investigation in confirming a diagnosis of PH is RHC, in which a catheter is inserted into the pulmonary artery via a vein in the groin or neck. RHC provides an accurate measurement of blood pressure in the pulmonary artery. Most patients suspected of having significant PH will undergo RHC.

After diagnosis of PH

Defining disease severity

Crucial to the management of patients with PH is an assessment of disease severity, which defines the prognosis and also helps to determine the most appropriate treatment. This assessment usually incorporates an assessment of symptoms (WHO functional class), exercise capacity (6 minute walk test, incremental shuttle walk test or cardio-pulmonary exercise testing [CPET]) and right ventricular function (echocardiography, MRI and RHC) (Galiè *et al.* 2009). CPET may be appropriate in patients with less severe forms of PH.

Follow-up assessments

Many of the tests and investigations used in the initial diagnosis of PH are also used during follow-up visits. PH is a life-long, incurable condition (with the exception of surgically resectable CTEPH), and regular follow-up visits are needed to monitor disease progression, effectiveness of treatment and quality of life. It is recommended that patients diagnosed with PAH and CTEPH and others treated with targeted drug therapy have routine follow-up appointments at a specialist PH centre (National PH Centres 2008). Investigations carried out may include exercise testing, echocardiography, ECG, CT or MRI scanning, and chest X-ray. RHC may also be repeated in some patients, including those on vasodilator therapy (calcium channel blockers) and those with an unclear clinical response to therapy.

Management and treatment of PH

The exact management and treatment a patient with PH will receive depends on the type of PH diagnosed. PAH and CTEPH are the only forms of PH for which specific treatment is available. PAH can be treated with targeted therapies. The treatment of choice for CTEPH in patients with potentially operable disease is pulmonary endarterectomy. In patients not suitable for pulmonary endarterectomy, targeted therapy may be beneficial (Galiè *et al.* 2009).

Targeted therapy used in PAH may be harmful in patients with PH due to left heart disease or lung disease (Hoeper *et al.* 2009). Treatment for these forms of PH usually concentrates on optimising treatment of the underlying condition. It is possible that a highly selected group of patients with severe PH in association with respiratory or left heart disease may benefit from targeted therapies but this requires further study.

The PH patient journey

A patient journey describes the patient's experience of a condition, from symptom onset through to living with the condition. It may include both the physical symptoms (such as effects on mobility) and the psychosocial effects such as the emotions associated with diagnosis and living with the condition (Armstrong *et al.* 2012, Flattery *et al.* 2005, Peloquin, Robichaud-Ekstran & Pepin 2007).

Each patient will have their own, individual patient journey, which will differ, depending on their illness and experiences. However, the patient journey can be broadly divided into the following sections:

- Pre-diagnosis (when the patient first notices symptoms)
- Diagnosis
- Treatment
- Living with the condition.

Why it is important to understand the patient journey

The patient journey can give healthcare workers an insight into many aspects of PH, including:

- The barriers and challenges a patient faces at different stages of the disease
- The factors that affect decision-making
- The interactions the patient has with healthcare professionals
- The emotional effects of PH

- Patients' attitudes and expectations (in terms of diagnosis, treatment and care)
- Variations in patients' adherence to medication
- The effects on family members, caregivers and others who are close to the patient
- The support the patient may need (practical, psychological, educational).

Living with PH

Living with PH presents several challenges. PH can have a profound effect on all aspects of a patient's life and the lives of those closest to them (Armstrong *et al.* 2012). This relates to the ability to carry out everyday tasks, the ability to work or attend education, and the emotions associated with having a serious life-limiting condition. Everyday tasks (such as shopping, doing the housework and even getting out of bed) can be difficult. Many patients have to give up work because of their illness, which further adds to the burden of PH.

Reflection point

PH is a rare disease and patients are often under the care of specialist PH centres. Consider some of the general factors involved in the assessment and management of the breathless patient and how these might be applied to the person with PH.

In 2010 the Pulmonary Hypertension Association (PHA UK) commissioned two pieces of research (The Impact Survey and The Lived Experience of PH) to try and understand the impact pulmonary arterial hypertension (PAH) has on patients and their caregivers, and what quality of life means to a patient with PAH. These two pieces of research provided invaluable insights into how PH impacts on the day-to-day lives of patients with the condition.

Once diagnosed with PH, patients are faced with the reality that it is a life-limiting condition (Armstrong *et al.* 2012). Dealing with this, and the uncertainty of prognosis, can lead to a range of issues for both patients and their family members and caregivers. These include dealing with the reality of having a terminal illness, including the practicalities of end of life, such as making a will, advanced care planning and funeral arrangements.

Healthcare professionals play an important role in ensuring that patients and family members have the support they need to address issues associated with end of life. Because prognosis for patients with PH is difficult to estimate and depends on a number of factors, end of life may need to be discussed when a patient is seemingly well. However, patients should be made aware of the unpredictability of their illness and the importance of thinking about end of life issues, regardless of the severity of their PH.

Targeted therapies as treatment for PH

PH can be treated using a range of different therapies. These include conventional (or supportive) therapies such as oxygen, warfarin and diuretics, and targeted drug therapies such as endothelin receptor antagonists (ambrisentan, bosentan), phosphodiesterase inhibitors (sildenafil, tadalafil) and prostaglandins (epoprostenol, iloprost, treprostinol). Patients are usually treated with a combination of conventional therapies and targeted drug therapies. Increasingly, patients receive more than one targeted drug therapy, although evidence for the effectiveness of combination therapy is still in its infancy.

CTEPH is another form of PH for which specific treatment is available. For these patients, a pulmonary endarterectomy can provide a potential cure. Pulmonary endarterectomy is an operation that can remove chronic clots from the lungs. However, some patients may not be suitable for pulmonary endarterectomy and may benefit instead from targeted drug therapies used in PH.

Oxygen therapy in PH management

While it is accepted that oxygen therapy is frequently used to treat patients with lung disease and hypoxaemia (particularly patients with COPD), there are no large studies of oxygen therapy in patients with PH or PAH. Studies have shown that oxygen therapy can reduce pulmonary vascular resistance in patients with PH that is associated with COPD. However, there are no randomised studies suggesting that long-term oxygen therapy is beneficial in PAH. There have been some small, uncontrolled studies that have reported improvements in patients with PAH who used supplemental oxygen. Oxygen therapy may therefore be beneficial to patients with PAH who are hypoxaemic.

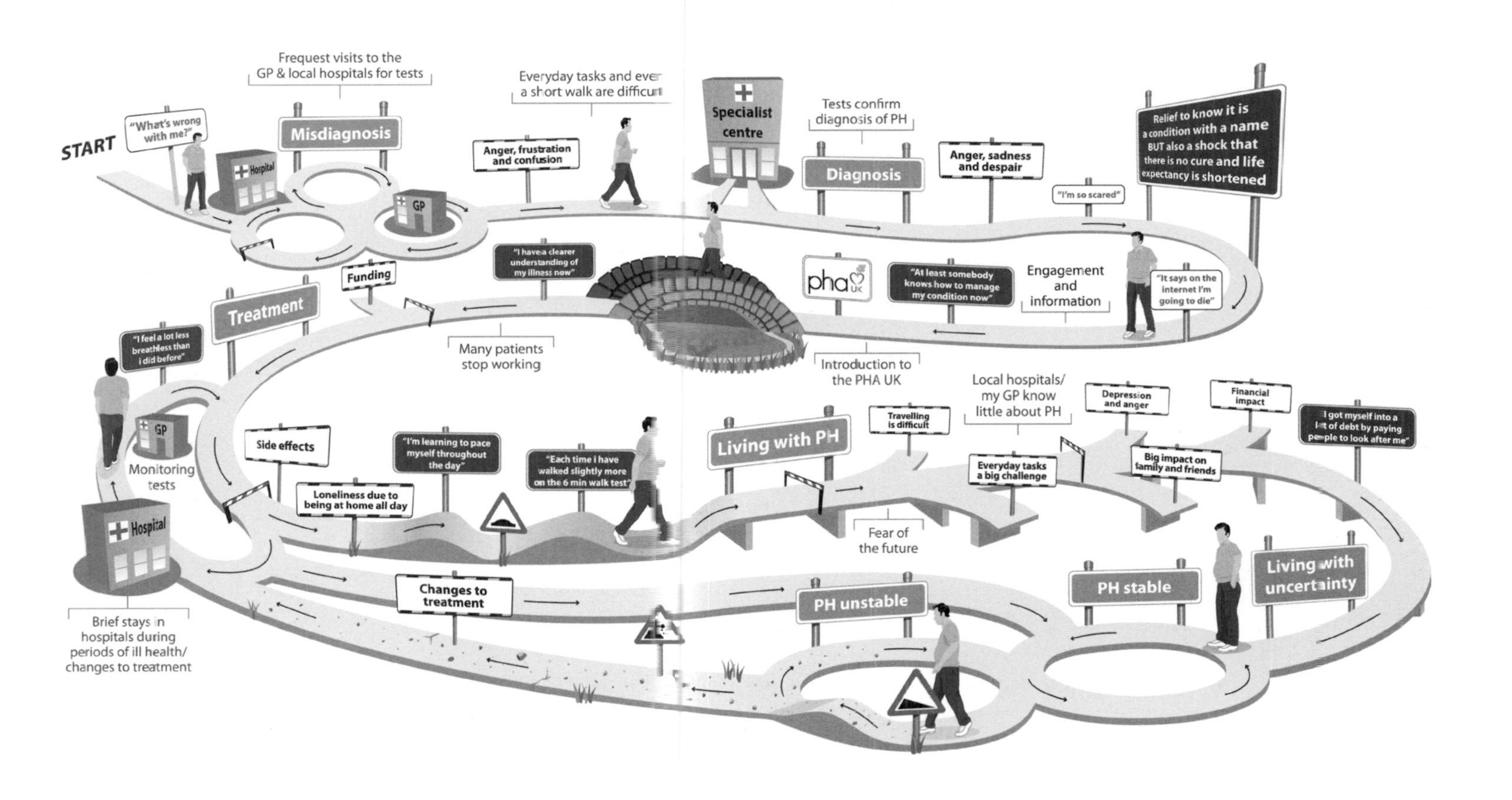

Figure 7.1: Pictorial representation of the patient's journey with PH

Source: Pulmonary Hypertension Association UK (www.phassociation.uk.com).

The goals of PH treatment

PH treatment is intended to:

- Improve the patient's symptoms
- Maintain or improve quality of life
- Prevent disease progression and extend survival.

It should be remembered that these goals often overlap with each other. In patients with PH, therapies that improve the blood flow through the lungs (by dilating the pulmonary arteries) will usually improve the function of the right heart and therefore extend patient survival. If more blood is pumped through the lungs, the patient will usually have fewer symptoms and a better quality of life. However, quality of life can also depend on the patient not having intolerable side effects from therapy.

Physical exertion for patients with pulmonary hypertension has typically been discouraged, due to cautiousness regarding oxygenation. However, evidence is emerging that participation in pulmonary rehabilitation is safe for patients with PH and may improve exercise capacity (Fox *et al.* 2011).

Summary

In conclusion, the diagnosis of pulmonary hypertension is often made at a mid to late stage in the course of the disease. From presentation, the majority of patients have an extended wait of around two years before they receive a final diagnosis. It is hoped that the advent of effective therapies and an increased awareness of the importance of early diagnosis and timely referral to specialist centres will improve the prognosis and quality of life for PH patients.

References

Armstrong, I., Rochnia, N., Harries, C., Bundock, S. & Yorke, J. (2012). The trajectory to diagnosis with pulmonary hypertension: a qualitative study. *British Medical Journal Open*. **2** (2): e000806. Published online 2012 April 18. doi: 10.1136/bmjopen-2011-000806.

Flattery, M.P., Pinson, J.M. & Savage, L. (2005). Living with pulmonary arterial hypertension: patients' experiences. *Heart Lung*. **34** (2), 99–107.

Fox, B.D., Kassirer, M., Weiss, I., Raviv, Y., Peled, N., Shitrit, D. & Kramer, M.R. (2011). Ambulatory rehabilitation improves exercise capacity in patients with pulmonary hypertension. *Journal of Cardiac Failure*. **17** (3), 196–200.

Galiè, N., Hoeper, M.M. & Humbert, M. (2009). Guidelines for the diagnosis and treatment of pulmonary hypertension. *European Heart Journal*. **34** (6), 1219–63.

Hoeper, M.M., Barberà, J.A. & Channick, R.N. (2009). Diagnosis, assessment and treatment of non-pulmonary arterial hypertension pulmonary hypertension. *Journal of the American College of Cardiology.* **54** (1), S85–96.

Humbert, M., Sitbon, O. & Chaouat, A. (2006). Pulmonary arterial hypertension in France. Results from a National Registry. *American Journal of Respiratory and Critical Care Medicine.* **173**, 1023–30.

McGoon, M., Gutterman, D. & Steen, V. (2004). Screening, early detection, and diagnosis of pulmonary arterial hypertension. ACCP evidence-based clinical practice guidelines. *Chest,* **126**, s14–34.

McGoon, M. & Kane, G. (2009). Pulmonary hypertension: diagnosis and management. *Mayo Clinical Proceedings.* **84**, 191–207.

McLaughlin, V., Archer, S.L. & Badesch, D.B. (2009). ACCF/AHA expert consensus document on pulmonary hypertension. A report of the American College of Cardiology Foundation Task Force on Expert Documents and the American Heart Association. *Journal of the American College of Cardiology,* **53**, 1573–619.

National Pulmonary Hypertension Centres of the UK and Ireland. (2008). Consensus statement on the management of pulmonary hypertension in clinical practice in the UK and Ireland. *Thorax.* **63** (Suppl ii), 1–41.

Peloquin. J., Robichaud-Ekstran, S. & Pepin J. (2007). Perception of quality of life by women with stage III or IV primary pulmonary hypertension and receiving treatment with prostacyclin. *Canadian Journal of Nursing Research.* **8**, 113e36.

Pulmonary Hypertension Association (PHA UK). (2010). The impact of living with pulmonary arterial hypertension. Results of two recent research projects commissioned by the Pulmonary Hypertension Association UK.

Simonneau, G., Robbins, I.M. & Beghetti, M.D. (2009). Updated clinical classification of pulmonary hypertension. *Journal of American College of Cardiology.* **54** (1), S43–54.

8

Non-pharmacological management of breathlessness

Julia Bott

Non-pharmacological management of breathlessness covers a broad spectrum of advice and interventions, from the purely physical (such as airway clearance techniques and exercise) to partially psychological (such as relaxation). Any non-pharmacological technique or strategy relies on a huge psychological component, since patients can choose to perform them or not, and as frequently or infrequently as they wish. The topic of psychological management is covered elsewhere.

Non-pharmacological management aims to alleviate symptoms and treat problems, rather than the disease itself. The goal is to maintain, restore or improve activity and/or function. It is above all about self-management, including lifestyle modifications: taking control of the disease to help reduce disability, thereby reducing the disease's impact and maximising participation in everyday life. Ultimately all the strategies discussed help alleviate breathlessness, even if that effect is not directly or necessarily obvious.

Non-pharmacological management is indicated in most respiratory conditions (Bauswein *et al.* 2008), but this discussion is restricted to its use in chronic disease. Strategies may be offered to groups and individuals, in the form of advice and education on self-management.

The full range of non-pharmacological strategies is listed below:

- Direct breathlessness management, including positioning and breathing techniques, walking aids and the use of hand-held fans
- Energy conservation techniques

- Airway clearance techniques
- Improvement or maintenance of mobility, physical activity and function
- Exercise prescription and training, including pulmonary rehabilitation (PR)
- The correct application of home oxygen therapy, including ambulatory oxygen
- Domiciliary non-invasive ventilation (NIV)
- Pain control and management
- Continence help and/or exercises
- Good nutrition and diet
- Smoking cessation
- Psychological help and support, including stress management.

Reflection point Reflection point Reflection point

Consider how many of the issues or strategies in the list above have you ever applied or considered referral for in the past, in the management of your breathless patients. Consider how you would get support with any of the above issues for a person in your care going forward.

This chapter will mainly focus on the first three strategies in the above list. Many of these strategies are full topics in themselves and beyond the remit of this chapter. Although the pain control and management techniques and continence help and exercises are likewise outside the scope of this chapter, they will be briefly touched on, as they need championing and they are frequently overlooked.

Energy conservation techniques will also be briefly covered, though not in depth. This area is usually the preserve of the occupational therapist (OT), who until 10 years ago was rarely seen in a respiratory service team. The input of OTs is invaluable (in terms of the physical and psychological aspects of the therapy they offer), whether in the acute or the community setting. It is advisable for an OT to gain some experience with a respiratory team in order to understand the particular needs of this client group and learn how energy conservation techniques need to be adapted in the light of altered respiratory mechanics.

Direct breathlessness management

Taking account of the altered mechanics of breathing is essential for effective positioning and use of the appropriate breathing exercises. The particular strategies adopted will depend on several factors – particularly on whether or not the patient has airway obstruction or a restrictive condition.

For patients with airway obstruction, such as chronic obstructive pulmonary disease (COPD) or asthma, the problem is hyperinflation of the chest, due to air being trapped as a result of the airways narrowing. Narrowed airways impede expiration, leaving *more* air than there should be at the end of expiration. Both functional residual capacity (FRC) and expiratory reserve volume (ERV) may increase, causing inspiratory capacity (IC) to reduce (West 2005a). This makes expiration harder, and the consequent hyperinflation forces the inspiratory muscles to adopt a 'permanently' shortened position, making it harder for them to generate power (due to a poor length–tension relationship) for the next inspiration.

Both these effects therefore increase the work required to breathe. The patient adopts a rapid, shallow breathing pattern, frequently with chest wall and abdominal asynchrony. There is reduced compliance, rendering it harder to breathe in against this increased resistance. (Think how hard it would be to force more air into a fully inflated balloon!) These changes may occur over a matter of years in COPD, and in a matter of hours or even minutes in an acute asthma attack. Either way, the strategy adopted needs to help improve the force-generating capacity of the inspiratory muscles and facilitate deflating the chest as much as possible during expiration.

For the individual with a restrictive condition, such as lung fibrosis, chest wall deformity or a neuromuscular condition, the problem is rather different. Here, the difficulty for the patient is under-inflation, since the disease has caused the lung to be constrained (restricted) during inspiration. This may be due to the lung tissue scarring and shrinking (caused by, for example, fibrosis or atelectasis), or to the deformity of the chest wall or weak inspiratory muscles. These individuals have a reduced FRC. In other words, there is *less* air left in the lung at the end of expiration than there should be (West 2005b). Either way, again, there is reduced compliance, making it harder to breathe in against this increased resistance. (Think of how hard it is blow up a completely deflated balloon.)

Positioning

Different body positions are used for a variety of purposes in respiratory care – for example, to improve ventilation/perfusion (V/Q) matching in the critically ill patient, or to use gravity to assist in clearing secretions (postural drainage). Either of these strategies may help reduce breathlessness when used appropriately, but the most common reason for positioning will be to help the patient minimise the detrimental effects of disturbed mechanics and altered muscle action (Green & Moxham 1983), and reduce the work of breathing and subsequent breathlessness.

For obstructive or restrictive problems, inspiration may need to be augmented by the accessory muscles of respiration (the upper fibres of the trapezius muscle and the sternocleidomastoid muscle). For instance, contraction of the upper fibres of the trapezius will usually bring about raising of the shoulders, and contraction of the sternocleidomastoid will turn the head. If these muscles are to function as muscles of respiration, they require the shoulder girdle to be 'fixed' (kept still), in order to allow them to reverse their usual action and help move the ribs instead.

Patients like to lean on something, because it brings about 'fixation'. However, if there is active fixation of the shoulder girdle (in other words, if they grip onto something), oxygen consumption is increased. They therefore need to be taught how to fix passively, without increasing oxygen consumption. Patients may be taught to lean their elbows on their knees (see Figure 8.1) or the arms of a chair, or a table when seated (see Figure 8.2), or on a suitable surface such as a windowsill or wall when standing (see Figure 8.3). When ambulating, they may find it helpful to rest their hands, or just thumbs, in or on their pockets (see Figure 8.4), belt loops, waistband or on an 'across the shoulder' handbag strap (see Figure 8.5) (Bott 2009, p.i9).

For the obstructed and hyperinflated patient, forward-leaning postures (see Figures 8.1, 8.2 and 8.3) improve the length–tension ratio of the diaphragm because the abdominal contents push up against the diaphragm and help it regain its domed position, which is more efficient for inspiration (Bott 2009, p.i10). In standing, the same principles apply, using hip flexion and therefore pelvic tilting, not spine flexion, to 'push' the abdominal contents into the pelvic cavity to load the diaphragm (see Figures 8.3, 8.4). This is why breathless patients like leaning on things, in order to utilise both shoulder girdle fixation and diaphragm loading.

For the person with a reduced FRC (that is, someone with less than the normal amount of air left in the lungs at the end of a tidal breath and whose diaphragm is therefore too domed or too high), the posture most likely to facilitate inspiration is upright sitting or standing (see Figure 8.6). This allows the abdominal contents to fall away from the pelvic cavity and the diaphragm can maximally descend, facilitating an increase in chest cage volume. Some patients find it helpful to wedge pillows (placed vertically) under their armpits, to elongate their thorax as much as possible to optimise this posture. It is imperative for all breathless patients (and especially those with lung restriction) to ensure that belts and waistbands are not tight, as they can impede abdominal motion and therefore diaphragmatic excursion. Think of women like Scarlett O'Hara in the film *Gone with the Wind*. Their corsets were so tight that they were forever having 'the vapours' – simply unable to breathe, due to restriction!

When it comes to lying down, again the patient needs to think about using the abdominal contents as a fulcrum for diaphragm loading. In other words, they should utilise the fact that the diaphragm will have more force in its descent if it can start in a domed position and has room to descend and flatten as it contracts. In side lying, the position of the lower limbs will influence this; the conventional 'recovery' position, with the uppermost (non-dependent) hip and knee flexed, 'unloads' the diaphragm. The abdominal contents will thus fall away, allowing unencumbered diaphragmatic excursion (see Figure 8.7). This position may be helpful in patients with restrictive problems and could be less useful for those with obstruction. In contrast, when the dependent (lowermost) hip and knee are flexed, this will tend to load' the diaphragm by pushing the abdominal contents inwards and therefore up on to the diaphragm, helping it to get into a more domed position. This may lead to improved respiratory muscle function in the patient with hyperinflation. As yet, studies have not been performed on patients in these positions to confirm the clinical effects of different lying and standing positions on the mechanics of breathing.

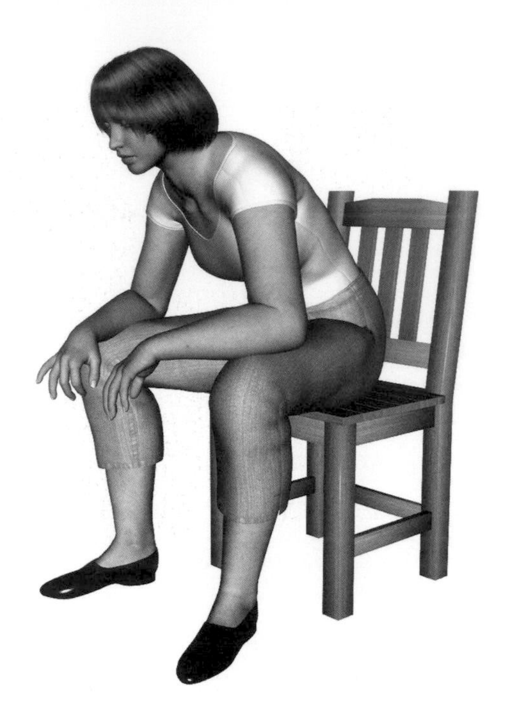

Figure 8.1:
Leaning elbows on knees

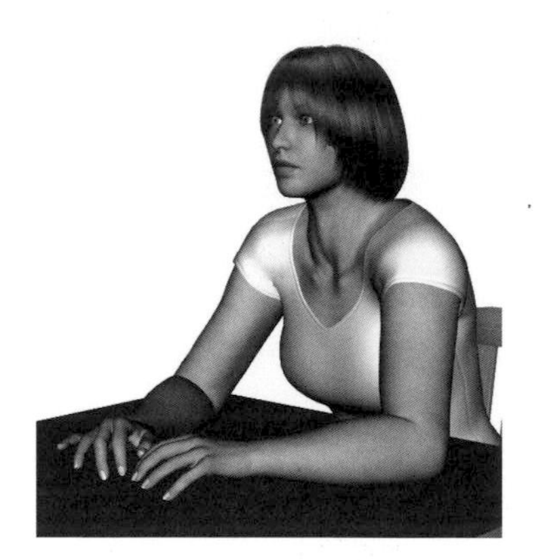

Figure 8.2:
Leaning elbows on table

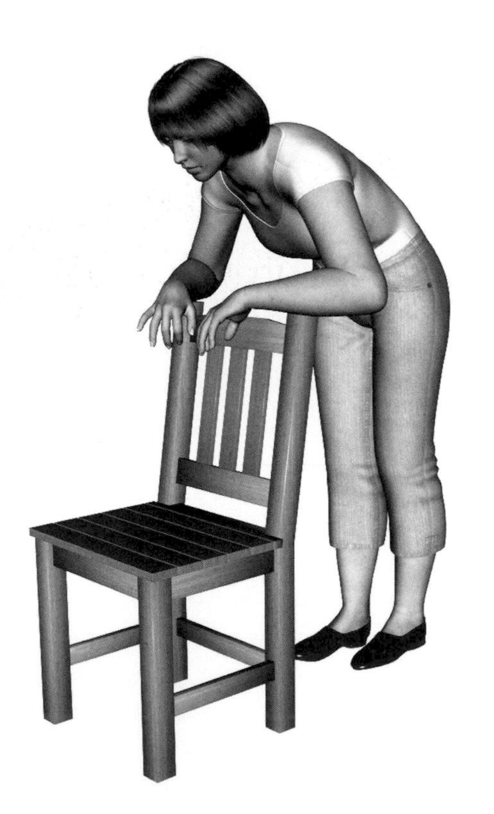

Figure 8.3:
Leaning elbows on a chair

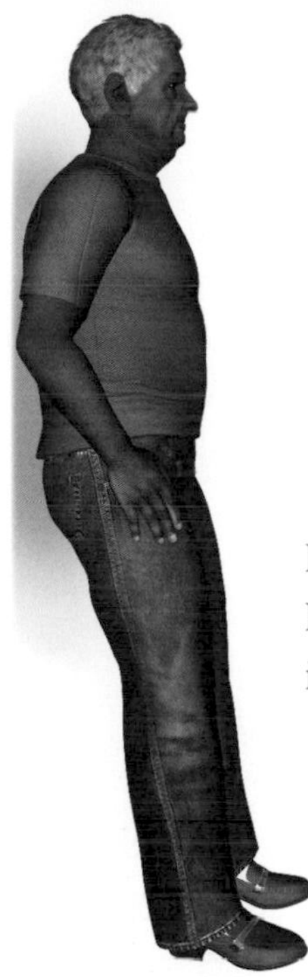

Figure 8.4:
Resting thumbs
in pocket

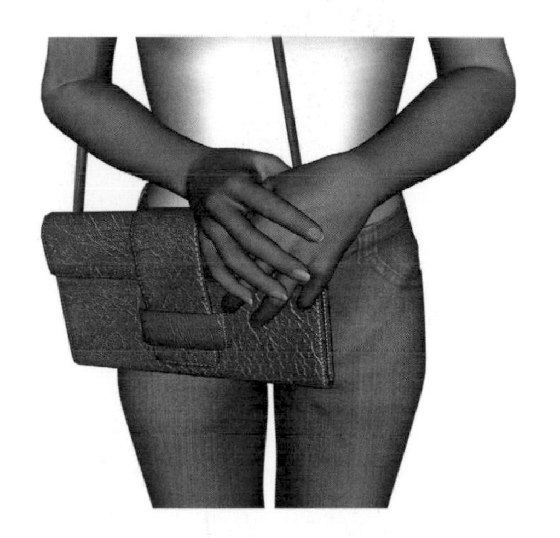

Figure 8.5:
Resting hands on
shoulder bag

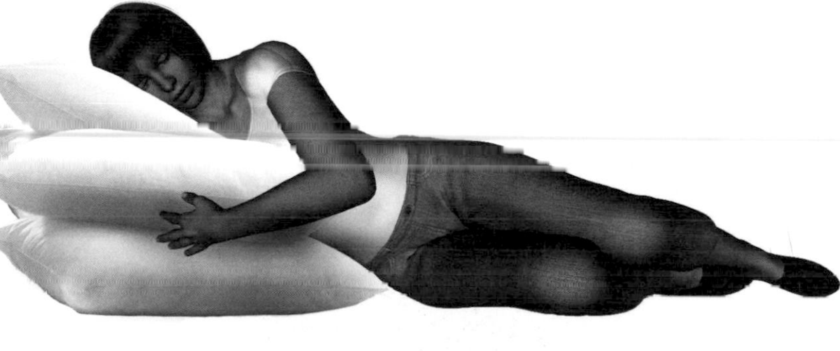

Figure 8.7:
Side lying

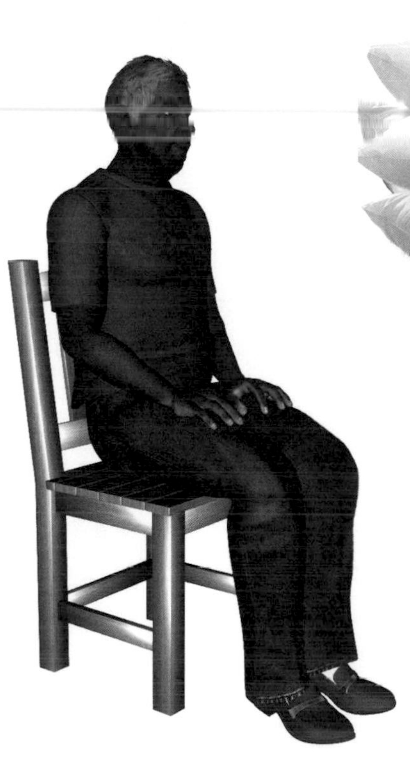

Figure 8.6:
Upright sitting

Walking aids

A wheeled walking aid (rollator frame) combines shoulder girdle fixation and forward-lean positioning. In COPD patients, it has been shown to reduce the ventilatory requirements of walking (Probst 2004). It is therefore particularly useful for those who are disabled by breathlessness and for those who use ambulatory oxygen. For the very disabled, a high, rollator frame will provide even more support (Yohannes 2003) and may, for example, allow a person to reach the toilet independently, rather than relying on assistance.

Breathing exercises

Breathing exercises and techniques can help the patient gain better control of their breathing, which can reduce both dyspnoea and panic. Techniques will vary, according to the underlying mechanics and whether the patient is at rest or undertaking exertion or exercise. Patients should be advised to practise the techniques that are right for them when they are well and at rest, so that they can be used when they are active and more likely to become breathless. Many of the techniques described below (Bott 2009, pp. i10–i11) can be combined effectively.

Breathing control

Breathing control means breathing gently, using the least possible effort, with arms supported and with the shoulders and hands relaxed. It is ideal to use in the forward-lean sitting position for those with COPD. Upright sitting (see Figure 8.6) may be preferred for those with lung restriction. The patient should be instructed to breathe gently and to try to relax and feel calmer with each exhalation. It is important not to confuse this with diaphragmatic breathing. Breathing control is suitable for any patient.

Diaphragmatic breathing

When a patient is breathless they are likely to breathe with the upper chest and shoulder muscles in a fast and shallow way – this can use up a lot of energy, make the person tire easily and make these muscles stiff and sore. An important aspect of managing breathlessness is learning a technique called controlled breathing (diaphragmatic breathing), which uses the diaphragm and lower chest muscles. Diaphragmatic breathing encourages excursion of the diaphragm, with passive outward motion of the abdominal wall (the abdominal contents being pushed forward by the descending diaphragm, not actively thrust out) and minimal chest wall movement. It can be encouraged by means of the therapist or patient placing a hand on the abdomen. This technique should not be used by those with hyperinflation. Although it may temporarily improve oxygen saturation, it can increase breathlessness in severe COPD patients, because greater effort is required to breathe due to poor mechanical efficiency. It is therefore not advisable to teach diaphragmatic breathing routinely to patients with severe COPD. However, this technique is very useful in asthma, hyperventilation syndrome and in restrictive conditions.

Steps to teach a patient diaphragmatic breathing:
Ask the patient to:

1. Get into a comfortable position – sitting with your neck, shoulders and back well supported – an upright chair with armrests or against a wall
2. Relax your shoulders, neck and arms
3. Place your hands on your tummy, just above your belly button
4. Give a little cough – the muscle you feel under your hand is your diaphragm
5. As you breathe in, allow your tummy to swell – you'll feel your hands rising and being pushed out by your diaphragm and tummy muscles
6. As you breathe out, relax and let your tummy fall.

Try and get a sense of breathing from around your waist rather than from your upper chest and feel your lungs expand as more air is able to get in.

Pursed-lip breathing

Pursed-lip breathing is thought to produce an increase in resistance to expiration, much like the positive expiratory pressure (PEEP) of airway clearance devices. Breathing against a partially closed mouth helps maintain back-pressure within the airways; this mechanism serves to support the alveoli and optimise gaseous exchange. The individual will usually have adopted this mechanism without being aware of its physiological implications (see Chapter 2). In fact, PEEP maintains pressure in the airway so that the lungs empty less completely in expiration, thus increasing the amount of air left in the lungs following expiration. This increases the pressure in the airways, helping to keep them open for longer and allowing expiration to be fuller, thus theoretically reducing ERV. It slows breathing rate and increases recovery rate when performed during exertion. It is therefore reasonable to teach pursed-lip breathing during exertion in patients with COPD. It has not been tested in patients with other conditions, but it is unlikely to benefit anyone without airway obstruction.

Exhalation on effort ('blow as you go')

'Blow as you go' is used to help the patient avoid inspiration during effort and breath-holding. Moving the shoulder girdle stops the muscles of the shoulder working as accessory muscles of respiration, so the load of breathing has to revert mainly to the diaphragm. This is why upper limb activities can markedly exacerbate dyspnoea. Inspiration itself also has an oxygen cost, since it is a high-energy activity for those with altered mechanics of breathing. For both these reasons, patients may have a tendency to breath-hold during exertion, which is counter-productive. To avoid these problems, the patient should be instructed to exhale when moving their shoulder girdle (for example, when lifting their arms above their head) or when stretching or lifting. They are also asked to exhale during effort that is difficult to combine with inspiration such as bending down or during the part of a movement involving the greatest effort – for instance, when standing up or stepping up. Breath-holding during any type of exertion should be strongly discouraged.

Relaxed, slower, deeper breathing

This is aimed at helping the patient avoid rapid shallow breathing, with subsequent inadequate alveolar ventilation, during exertion. Over 30 years ago it was demonstrated that slow, controlled breathing to a pre-determined speed produced an increase in tidal volume and a reduction in the arterial partial pressure of carbon dioxide ($PaCO_2$). Another study, however, suggested that this pattern of breathing may predispose to fatigue of the diaphragm when the expiratory time was then shortened, so the technique is advocated in combination with techniques to increase length of expiration (pursed lips breathing and 'blow-as-you-go'). It must be stressed that the change in rate and depth are in relation only to the patient's own natural pattern. The use of a pulse oximeter during exertion and tests of exercise tolerance are useful indicators of the efficacy of the technique. This technique is not advocated for an acutely breathless patient and its use is best confined to activity.

Paced breathing

This technique has similar aims to slow, relaxed breathing and is also used during exertion to reduce dyspnoea – for example, when climbing the stairs or walking. It helps avoid rushing, breath-holding or rapid shallow breathing. The patient is instructed to inhale and exhale in time with steps, in a rhythm that suits them. It utilises a combination of the other techniques to suit the activity and the individual.

Using hand-held fans

For some years there have been reports of breathlessness being palliated by applying a cold stimulus towards the cheek. Some of the perceived (placebo) effect of oxygen therapy in those who are not hypoxaemic is probably due to this, rather then the oxygen itself. In a randomised controlled trial, cold air blowing against the cheek significantly reduced breathlessness when normal subjects breathed against an inspiratory resistive load until hypercapnia was induced (Schwartzstein *et al.* 1987). The same effect was not observed when cold air was directed to their legs.

In contrast, no difference was found between a hand-held fan and wristbands in a two-month trial in 70 patients with severe breathlessness due to end-stage disease (Bausewein *et al.* 2010). By the end of the study data were available on only 24 patients in the hand-held fan group, and 12 in the wristband group, due to large drop-out rate and death. Around 50% of the patients were still using the hand-held fan, compared with only 20% using the wristband. However, there is currently not enough data to judge the evidence for a variety of non-pharmacological techniques, including fan therapy (Bausewein *et al.* 2008). Many patients report finding a fan helpful, and it can be used to help wean non-hypoxaemic patients off oxygen, or to reduce the inspired fraction of oxygen in those who like the high flow but do not clinically need it.

Energy conservation techniques

Energy conservation is aimed at minimising the work of activities of daily living (ADL). This enables the patient to save energy on doing the tasks they *have* to do, and allow some for those they *want* to do. It is commonly taught within pulmonary rehabilitation units but may also be taught on an individual basis, ideally by an occupational therapist. The techniques help reduce the energy expended in performing a task by using organisation and pacing of tasks and alternative ways to undertake them. This may mean changing posture to allow forward leaning or upright sitting (as required by the patient's altered respiratory mechanics), or fixing the shoulder girdle while undertaking tasks of the upper limb (such as shaving or hair brushing), or sitting down to do simple chores, such as washing up, thereby using less energy.

Energy conservation also includes appropriate use of home adaptations, such as a seat or hand rail, lowering or raising of objects, or the use of small aids to reduce or eliminate high effort movement, such as a 'helping hand' to reach for high objects, or a 'sock aid' to put on socks. One small study showed a statistically significant benefit on dyspnoea of energy conservation techniques used during standardised activities of daily living (Velloso & Jardim 2006). Pragmatically, it is sensible to combine energy conservation techniques with the breathing techniques described earlier.

Airway clearance techniques

The use of airway clearance techniques has been documented for over a century; postural drainage for secretion removal in bronchiectasis was described as long ago as 1901. Several airway clearance techniques are now available and this allows patients to better manage their secretions in a way that suits them. Regrettably postural drainage has fallen out of fashion, with healthcare professionals assuming that it is outmoded or has been superseded by newer techniques. However, the correct technique should always be carefully chosen to suit the condition and the patient, and its efficacy assessed (Bott *et al.* 2009, p. i15).

Possible techniques include:

- Independent techniques requiring no equipment and using a variety of breathing exercises; the Active Cycle of Breathing Techniques (ACBT) and Autogenic Drainage (AD).
- Small, hand-held devices to deliver positive expiratory pressure (PEP) or oscillating PEP, frequently used in conjunction with one of the above, or specific elements of them.
- Postural drainage or modified postural drainage. Although postural drainage is rarely indicated in non-suppurative chest disorders, its efficacy should be assessed in every patient with non-cystic fibrosis (CF)

bronchiectasis, since it has been shown to increase airway clearance in this client group. Modified postural drainage is used more specifically for patients with CF and occasionally for those with other conditions, such as COPD, where there are large volumes of secretions and these are amenable to the effects of gravity. There are specific contraindications to postural drainage where there is risk attached to a person having their head lower than their body and/or legs.

- Large mechanical devices that either encompass the whole thorax (such as high-frequency chest wall oscillation jackets) or provide pressurised airflow via tubing and a mouthpiece or mask (such as cough-assist machines). These are indicated more specifically for patients with very hard-to-clear secretions, such as the thick, tenacious secretions of CF, or where the problem is lack of muscle power to perform the cough, as in chest wall or neuromuscular disorders or diseases.
- Nebulised substances (such as bronchodilators, saline or hypertonic saline), which, when used prior to one of the airway clearance techniques, can enhance its effect.

It is important to appreciate that finding the correct technique may take time; not all patients or problems will suit all techniques, since sputum rheology varies markedly between patients and between conditions, and some techniques are contraindicated in specific situations or may have unwanted side effects. Moreover, patient preference and likely adherence to therapy must be included in the decision algorithm. Training in the pathophysiology of the diseases, and subsequent alterations in both sputum and mucociliary escalator function, as well as in all the techniques is essential, to ensure airway clearance is both optimally and safely addressed.

Physical activity, exercise prescription and training, including cardiac and pulmonary rehabilitation

Exercises for pulmonary problems were first recorded for patients with chest injuries in 1915, but conventionally many tuberculosis (TB) sanatoria and hospitals provided physical exercises, often in the fresh air, as part of their treatment. For many patients and some healthcare professionals, it seems counter-intuitive to ask a very breathless person to be active or to exercise.

However, it is actually lack of activity and exercise that leads to de-conditioning (muscle weakening and atrophy), which in turn increases oxygen requirement, breathlessness, and fear of activity and exertion, along with a host of other negative effects. This is known as 'the vicious cycle of inactivity'. The inability to walk far is a strong predictor of mortality. The very act of exercising brings about very beneficial results, since strong muscles require less oxygen to work than weak ones, the body becomes more flexible, joints will be stimulated to secrete synovial fluid to lubricate movement and all this makes movement more efficient and reduces breathlessness. Cardiac and pulmonary rehabilitation have a wealth of evidence demonstrating the beneficial effects of exercise and this can be delivered at home or at a rehabilitation centre (Nici *et al.* 2006, Dalal *et al.* 2010).

Physical activity and exercise should therefore be encouraged for all patients with a chronic pulmonary condition throughout the course of their disease, including during and post-exacerbation, as well as during hospital admission where possible and appropriate (Puhan *et al.* 2005). Exercise training programmes, including rehabilitation, are indicated for patients who have symptoms and impaired physical activities in daily life. Exercise is most effective when supervised by a healthcare professional skilled in the delivery of exercise prescription and training. Exercise should always be prescribed at an appropriate intensity for that individual, since higher-intensity training produces a greater effect and the correct prescription requires careful assessment. Selected patients may benefit from inspiratory muscle training (O'Brien *et al.* 2008).

Musculo-skeletal dysfunction and pain

Many individuals with chronic cardiac and respiratory conditions suffer from co-existent pain. This may be due to co-morbidity, such as osteoarthritis of the spine or knees, or to osteoporosis, but may also be as a direct consequence of the respiratory condition, due to poor posture and/or poor flexibility and inactivity. Joints that are not regularly moved through their full range cease to produce adequate synovial fluid, leading to pain and stiffness, which then inhibits movement. This starts a vicious cycle of inactivity, compounding the existing one due to the breathlessness. With increasing years too, the likelihood of such problems increases, as does the prevalence of foot problems, which also inhibit activity and increase de-conditioning, compounding breathlessness. Patients should be asked (as part of a thorough respiratory assessment) about the presence of any musculo-skeletal pain. If present, they should be referred to an appropriate service, such as podiatry or specialist musculo-skeletal physiotherapy.

Continence help and/or exercises

Stress incontinence may indirectly make breathlessness worse, since it is likely to inhibit performance of forced expiratory manoeuvres, such as coughing and spirometry or physical exertion, and therefore impact on adherence/compliance with self-management strategies. As there is an increased prevalence of stress incontinence in those with a chronic cough due to CF, and as incontinence is worse in those with COPD and CF (compared with a normal population with stress incontinence), its presence or absence should be ascertained by sensitive questioning in every patient with a chronic cough. If present, a referral to a physiotherapist specialising in this field is warranted, since significant improvements can often be made through use of the appropriate pelvic floor exercises (Button *et al.* 2005). If ongoing support or management of persistent incontinence is needed, then referral on to a continence nurse should be considered.

Summary

All too frequently, the phrase 'self-management' is used to describe simple action plans for inhaler use during exacerbation, whereas patients who are breathless should really be offered a wide range of non-pharmacological techniques to support them in managing their disease and their symptoms. This is true self-management. The choice of which techniques to use will depend on the stage of the disease, the symptoms and the mechanical derangement underlying the symptoms. Most of the techniques outlined in this chapter should be covered in a good pulmonary rehabilitation course and this is one of the many reasons why PR should be offered to all appropriate patients. The sooner a patient with a chronic lung condition learns these useful 'tools' to help their symptoms and, in some cases, reduce disease and symptom progression, the better their self-management will be.

References

Bausewein, C., Booth, S., Gysels, M. & Higginson, I. (2008). Non-pharmacological interventions for breathlessness in advanced stages of malignant and non-malignant diseases. The Cochrane Library, 2.

Bausewein, C., Booth, S., Gysels, M., Kühnbach, R. & Higginson, I. (2010). Effectiveness of a hand-held fan for breathlessness: a randomised phase II trial. *BMC Palliative Care*. **9**, 22.

Bott, J., Blumenthal, S., Buxton, M. & Ellum, S. (2009). Guidelines for the physiotherapy management of the adult, medical, spontaneously breathing patient. *Thorax*. **64** (suppl1) i1–i51.

Button, B.M., Sherburn, M., Chase, J., Stillman, B. & Wilson, J. (2005). Effect of a three months physiotherapeutic intervention on incontinence in women with chronic cough related to cystic fibrosis and COPD. *Pediatric Pulmonology*. **40**, a369.

Dalal, H.M., Zawada, A., Jolly, K., Moxham, T. & Taylor, R.S. (2010). Home based versus centre based cardiac rehabilitation: Cochrane systematic review and meta-analysis. *British Medical Journal*. **340**, b5631

Green, M. & Moxham, J. (1983). 'Respiratory muscles in health and disease' in Barnes, P. (ed.) *Respiratory Medicine: Recent Advances*. Fenley DC, Petty TL. Butterworth Heinemann pp.1–20.

Holloway, E.A. & West, R. (2007). Integrated breathing and relaxation training (the Papworth Method) for adults with asthma in primary care: a randomised controlled trial. *Thorax*. **62**, 1039–42.

O'Brien, K., Geddes, E.L., Reid, W.D., Brooks, D. & Crowe, J. (2008). Inspiratory muscle training compared with other rehabilitation interventions in chronic obstructive pulmonary disease: a systematic review update. *Journal of Cardiopulmonary Rehabilitation*. **28**, 128–41.

Nici, L., Donner, C., Wouters, E., Zuwallack, R., Ambrosino, N., Bourbeau, J., Carone, M., Celli, B., Engelen, M., Fahy, B., Garvey, C., Goldstein, R. & Gosselink, R. (2006). American Thoracic Society/European Respiratory Society statement on pulmonary rehabilitation. *American Journal of Respiratory and Critical Care Medicine*. **173**, 1390–413.

Probst, V.S., Troosters, T., Coosemans, I., Spruit, M.A., Pitta Fde, O., Decramer, M. & Gosselink, R. (2004). Mechanisms of improvement in exercise capacity using a rollator in patients with COPD. *Chest*. **126**, 1102–7.

Puhan, M.A., Scharplatz, M., Troosters, T. & Steurer, J. (2005). Respiratory rehabilitation after acute exacerbation of COPD may reduce risk for readmission and mortality – a systematic review. *Respiratory Research*. **6** (1), 54.

Schwartzstein, R.M., Lahive, K., Pope, A., Weinberger, S.E. & Weiss, J.W. (1987). Cold facial stimulation reduces breathlessness induced in normal subjects. *American Review of Respiratory Disease*. **136** (1), 58–61.

Velloso, M. & Jardim, J.R. (2006). Study of energy expenditure during activities of daily living using and not using body position recommended by energy conservation techniques in patients with COPD. *Chest*. **130**, 126–32.

West, J.B. (2005a). *Obstructive Diseases in Pulmonary Pathophysiology – The Essentials*. (7th edn) Philadelphia, US: Lippincott Williams & Wilkins, pp. 49–80.

West, J.B. (2005b). *Restrictive Diseases in Pulmonary Pathophysiology – The Essentials*. (7th edn) Philadelphia, US: Lippincott Williams & Wilkins, pp. 81–98.

Yohannes, A.M. & Connolly, M.J. (2003). Early mobilization with walking aids following hospital admission with acute exacerbation of chronic obstructive pulmonary disease. *Clinical Rehabilitation*. **17**, 465–71.

9

Psychological strategies to manage breathlessness

Jessica Callaghan

The prevalence of anxiety and depression in patients with cardiac and respiratory disease is higher than in the general population and it is well accepted that psychological factors impact on quality of life, use of healthcare resources and self-management (Lingen 2007; Maurer *et al.* 2008, Yohannes *et al.* 2010). Even in those patients who do not experience symptoms of anxiety or depression, the adjustment to reduced function and independence is psychologically demanding. In addition to this, as already discussed in previous chapters, the experience of breathlessness can be distressing in itself.

In this chapter we will consider the following non-pharmacological approaches, which address the *psychological* impact of breathlessness:

- Psychoeducation
- Cognitive Behavioural Therapy principles and treatment approaches
- Distraction techniques
- Social support and activity
- Lifestyle balance and restructuring
- Relaxation techniques
- Mindfulness
- Motivation and barriers to change.

All professions working with this client group have a lot to offer if psychological approaches can be embedded into usual practice. However, a community team will benefit greatly from the contribution of an occupational therapist (OT), psychologist or counsellor with psychological training and experience. One or more of these professionals would ideally be based within a specialist team and would be able to develop their knowledge of respiratory or cardiac conditions so that the psychological support becomes a seamless part of service provision. However, this opportunity rarely arises, and generalist psychological services are more often used. If funding is available for such a role, be aware that each profession will bring their own style of treatment and so the needs of the client group and team must always be considered.

All psychological interventions (whoever they are delivered by) are best used in conjunction with the physical and practical strategies outlined in Chapter 8, as these build self-efficacy ('I can cope with breathlessness; I know what to do') and restore a sense of control, which in turn helps to counteract the anxiety–breathlessness spiral.

Active listening skills are key to understanding the psychological aspects of the patient's breathlessness experience. This understanding will aid assessment and individualised treatment planning, maximise the chance of adherence, and strengthen the therapeutic relationship, which can have a significant impact on treatment outcomes (Hall *et al.* 2010). Whilst we can expect common themes in the patient's experience of breathlessness according to their diagnosis (as explored by Gysels & Higginson 2011), we must recognise that a unique set of experiences and belief systems underpin the psychological response to breathlessness for that individual.

The most commonly researched psychological interventions for anxiety and depression in chronic illness are cognitive and behavioural interventions, problem-solving techniques, relaxation and miscellaneous stress management interventions (Coventry *et al.* 2013). Most studies have been in the field of chronic obstructive pulmonary disease (COPD). The COPD literature supports psychological interventions in conjunction with exercise, but there is a lack of evidence for their use as stand-alone treatments. However, national guidelines developed in the UK support the identification of anxiety and depression, and point us towards Cognitive Behavioural Therapy (CBT)-based interventions for patients who have a long-term condition with co-existing anxiety and/or depression.

Assessment of the psychological impact of breathlessness

Initial assessment

If you want to assess anxiety or depression within an already time-restricted physical assessment (see Chapter 3), key questions need to relate to whether breathlessness *causes* and/or *is caused by* anxiety, and whether low mood is a problem for the patient. You need to know to what extent anxiety and depression are affecting daily functioning in order to understand the severity of the problem. In addition to the screening questions suggested by the relevant NICE guidelines (see boxes below), you may find it useful to use the Patient Health Questionnaire (Gilbody *et al.* 2007) and the Generalised Anxiety Disorder Scale (Spitzer *et al.* 2006). Information gained can be used when feeding back to the patient and GP. Some quality-of-life measures will also give information about how breathlessness is affecting the individual's confidence, social functioning and general coping.

Other factors to consider when assessing the psychological impact of breathlessness, include:

- History of breathlessness linking with emotions
- Trigger situations and examples of breathlessness
- Stressful, anxious or angry thoughts bringing on breathlessness even when there is no exertion
- Experience of loss (roles, routines, relationships that have changed)
- Level of social support
- Activities or situations they now avoid because of breathlessness
- Stresses other than health-related ones, e.g. accommodation, relationship or financial stresses
- Ways in which they try to control breathlessness/anxiety/low mood spirals
- Level of awareness of how emotions and breathlessness affect each other.

During an assessment, you can gain a lot of information through observation, careful listening and gentle probing about insight, self-awareness, self-efficacy and motivation to change. All of these have the potential to influence people's response to non-pharmacological treatments.

1 'Depression in adults with a chronic physical health problem: Treatment and management' (NICE 2009)

The NICE guidelines suggest asking about two main features of depression:

1. **A sense of hopelessness**, sadness or low mood. This may include being tearful.
2. **A loss of interest or pleasure**. It is often the spouse or relative who mentions something the patient always used to enjoy (e.g. doing the crossword, or watching the grandchildren play) but no longer enjoys.

If these two symptoms are present, then you need to enquire about other symptoms of depression, such as:

- Disturbed sleep (decreased or increased compared to usual)
- Decreased or increased appetite and/or weight
- Fatigue
- Agitation
- Poor concentration
- Feelings of worthlessness or guilt
- Suicidal thoughts.

2 'Assessment of Generalised Anxiety Disorder' (NICE 2011)

The NICE guidelines suggest asking about two main features of generalised anxiety disorder:

1. **Excessive anxiety and worry** about different life stresses.
2. **Problems controlling worrying thoughts** – feeling like this most days.

If these two symptoms are present, then you need to enquire about other symptoms of anxiety, such as:

- Being restless
- Fatigue
- Poor concentration
- Frequently feeling irritable
- Muscle tension
- Problems sleeping.

Panic attacks

Some patients will describe a breathlessness attack and it can be difficult to tell whether it is purely physical, a panic attack or a mixture of the two. Many patients do not know the difference, and being able to ask questions to help determine this is important for the patient's sense of control and for treatment planning. It can be useful to observe the patient when they are breathless in order to determine how much of the breathlessness is panic related (see Box 2, above, for some suggestions as to what to look for).

In practice, the defining symptom that most commonly indicates panic for this patient group is 'a feeling of impending doom' and this is accompanied by some very strong physical symptoms (obviously the increased respiratory rate but they may also have palpitations, shaking and sweating). There are often specific fears underlying the panic such as 'I won't ever get control of this breathing' or 'I'm going to have a heart attack'.

Patients with interstitial lung disease often present with a panting breathing pattern. The fast respiratory rate may look similar to panic breathlessness so you should always ask the patient if they are aware of having anxious thoughts or feeling worried.

Also, be mindful of hyperventilation syndrome, which can mean that the patient has an unusual breathing pattern in addition to their cardiac or respiratory condition. Hyperventilation syndrome symptoms mean that the patient will tip into panic more easily. However, the dysfunctional breathing pattern can be treated and changed if the patient is self motivated (Bott *et al.* 2009).

Anticipatory anxiety

Anticipatory anxiety is a significant problem for the breathless patient, as it is often the main reason for avoidance behaviours and inactivity. The patient anticipates how breathless a task will make them, and begins to experience breathlessness at the *thought* of moving. This in turn makes them even less likely to get up (out of their safe, comfortable place) and carry out a particular task.

Depression

In the breathless patient, low mood can initially be hidden. You may ask about low mood because of symptoms or behaviours you notice over a period of time, such as lack of motivation, reduced eye contact, lethargy or passive responses. The spouse or relative may comment on a lack of appetite or irritability. Dysthymia (low-level depression that continues for several years) is sometimes present and can be particularly difficult to treat – see Box 1 (page 132) for some suggestions as to what to look for.

Reflection point Reflection point Reflection point

When assessing how much of the person's breathlessness is panic, you should consider the following questions:

- Is the patient aware of feeling anxious or stressed?
- What language does the patient use about breathlessness?
- Is the breathlessness disproportionate or inconsistent?
- Is there shortness of breath prior to exertion (anticipatory anxiety)?
- Is there an increased respiratory rate when discussing stressful topics?
- Is the patient showing avoidance or reassurance-seeking behaviours?

Also consider: psychiatric history, current life stresses, recovery time, posture at rest and on exertion, breathing pattern.

Psychoeducation

Whilst any educational input must be individualised (tailored to the patient's condition, level of understanding and educational level), there are certain topics that can usefully be considered in relation to breathlessness.

Physical symptoms versus anxiety and depression

Firstly, the symptoms of the physical condition need to be differentiated from the common symptoms of anxiety and depression. An anxious or depressed person may easily misinterpret their symptoms and can be very sensitive to any changes in their body. If they know what to expect (and which symptoms can be attributed to their physical condition, and which to anxiety or depression), a great deal of uncertainty and associated fear can be removed. For some patients, this will be enough to control the mild panic episodes that were previously triggered by, for example, exertion-related breathlessness. Providing education about the breathlessness spirals (inactivity, anxiety, depression, social isolation) will also help to normalise these reactions and can be reassuring and improve insight.

The adrenalin response

The patient needs to understand the adrenalin response so that they understand how their respiratory rate can be affected by anxious thoughts. Ask the patient to consider examples of what makes them breathless and what makes them feel stressed, anxious or angry. It may be that breathlessness from exertion makes them anxious (and triggers the adrenalin response), or that thinking about a stressful event or situation makes them breathless (due to the increased respiratory rate caused by the adrenalin response). Ask the patient to identify what physical symptoms they usually get when feeling anxious or stressed. Explain the fight/flight response and then explain the physiological reason for each of their symptoms. This will help remove fear of the physical symptoms (such as palpitations) and can stop the anxiety spirals being fuelled by fear of the adrenalin response itself. Remember that the physiological response in the body is the same for anger as for anxiety.

Taking education to the next level and assisting patients in identifying their usual patterns of thoughts/symptoms/behaviours is the first step towards a CBT-based intervention (see below).

Reflection point

It's all about the language...

Consider the language you use when discussing the emotional aspects of breathlessness. Mirror the patient's language where possible, but if it is an initial assessment consider using the following terms:

- 'Feeling low' rather than 'depression'
- 'Worried' rather than 'anxious'
- 'Frustration' rather than 'anger'
- 'Breathlessness attack' rather than 'panic attack' (until you have established the balance between exertion breathlessness and panic in trigger situations).

Once the patient begins to open up and if you suspect a problem with any of the above, then using stronger language can be useful and may be an important part of psychoeducation.

Psychological loss and adjustment

Patients with chronic conditions will experience an increasing sense of psychological loss relating to activities, roles and routines that used to give structure and quality to their lives. The effect on relationships can be challenging, and an individual's sense of their own identity can be shaken when their role as a husband, wife, worker, parent or friend is under threat – particularly if they feel unable to fulfil these roles to meet their own or others' expectations. It can be useful to consider *adjustment* as a more helpful term than *acceptance*, as with progressive disease the patient continually has to adjust and adapt (Pierobon 2011). Drawing a parallel with a bereavement response can also be useful, in order to explain the possible progression of emotions and responses they may experience (Denial, Anger, Bargaining, Depression and Acceptance), the 'five stages of grief' identified by the psychiatrist Elisabeth Kübler-Ross in her books (Kübler-Ross 1969, 2005). However, you should also be sure to explain that these stages are rarely experienced in a linear way.

Using Cognitive Behaviour Therapy (CBT) principles

CBT involves identifying thinking and behaviour patterns and changing the ones that are unhelpful. Most evidence-based rehabilitation programmes for patients with chronic conditions are underpinned by CBT principles. For example in pulmonary rehabilitation (PR), psychological and social support provided within pulmonary rehabilitation settings can facilitate adjustment by encouraging adaptive thoughts and behaviours, helping patients to diminish negative emotions, and providing a socially supportive environment (Nici *et al.* 2006). CBT principles can also be used in individual work and can enable health professionals to understand why a patient may respond well to the teaching of non-pharmacological strategies, or struggle to benefit from these strategies.

The five areas approach to CBT (Williams & Garland 2002) allows visual mapping of the interaction between the patient's thoughts and behaviours in a specific situation (see Figure 9.1 below). It may be helpful to write notes in the different sections as the patient is describing a situation, prompting them as necessary so that all sections are filled in. Then, looking at the diagram together, you can ask the patient which aspects link with each other and use arrows to indicate the direction. Arrows usually go everywhere, which is a useful visual demonstration of the close links between thoughts, feelings, physical symptoms and actions/behaviours. You can also use it to make the point that the whole process usually starts with a thought, even if a physical symptom is what the patient first becomes aware of. This helps patients understand how physical symptoms create further worrying thoughts, and that some actions may be helpful while others are unhelpful. In my experience, even people who seem to have very little insight benefit from this awareness-raising exercise. It also assists the health professional in their assessment and can help the patient understand why it is useful to try the wide range of practical, cognitive and behavioural strategies available.

Nevertheless, not everyone will benefit from a CBT approach. For example, someone who cannot concentrate or engage (due to pain or severe depression) will experience limited benefit.

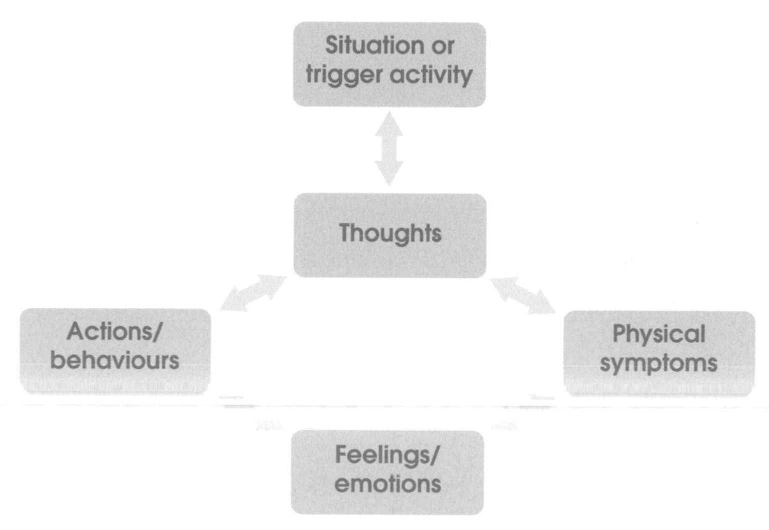

Figure 9.1: The five areas approach model.
Adapted from Williams, C. & Garland, A. (2002).

Problem-solving

Breathlessness, fear and loss of confidence can make clear thinking and decision-making difficult. Similarly, problem-solving can become harder. The aim is to build the patient's problem-solving skills so that they can face problem situations or triggers for breathlessness, and be able to 'step back' psychologically. They may need to take time to understand a problem and their response, and consider any solutions there may be. Solutions may be practical and involve energy conservation strategies (such as breaking an activity into manageable sections), or there may be a cognitive solution such as viewing a situation in a different way. The health professional can assist a patient in the process of reflecting back and analysing a breathlessness event or problem situation. The aim is to differentiate between those aspects of the problem that can be changed, and those that cannot be changed and have to be faced (or viewed in a different way) in order to restore a sense of control or adjustment. Livermore (2010) studied the effect of a brief CBT intervention for COPD patients, which included problem-solving to reduce barriers to effective coping. The group using the CBT intervention showed a reduction in panic attacks and levels of anxiety and depression, compared with the routine care group.

Identifying unhelpful thoughts

Identifying negative or unhelpful thinking patterns can be difficult – even for those patients with good insight. However, health professionals can become very skilled at drawing out key negative or anxious thoughts from a conversation, and using these as a basis for further questioning.

Here is an example of this approach being used with a patient who is avoiding showering because of the breathlessness–anxiety spiral:

> 'When you were describing that panic attack in the shower, you said you felt so bad you thought you were going to have a heart attack. Do you think this is at the root of your anxiety in the shower?'
>
> 'Is there anything else that worries you about showering?'
>
> 'What other thoughts go through your mind?'
>
> 'What do you fear most about showering?'

As the patient talks, you can write down the content of those worrying thoughts, identifying how a question such as 'what if I have a heart attack and no one finds me?' can turn into the corresponding negative belief 'when I have a shower I may have a heart attack and die alone'. Any interpretation you make needs to be checked with the patient; collaborative working helps identify specific thoughts, which can then be used to develop coping thoughts. Before moving on to the coping thought, you can teach the patient about thinking distortions that occur when we feel anxious or low. (It is helpful to explain that we are all susceptible to such patterns of thinking, given certain experiences or conditions.) Common thinking distortions include:

- 'All or nothing' ('black and white') thinking (either 'really well' or 'terrible', either 'coping completely' or 'not coping at all')
- 'Over-generalising' ('nothing ever goes right for me' or 'I am never in control of my breathing')
- Jumping to conclusions ('I won't get any benefit from pulmonary rehabilitation – there's no point in going').

If the patient has clinical anxiety or depression, unhelpful thinking styles can become more frequent, last longer and be more intense, intrusive and believable. Consequently the vicious thought–behaviour cycles become reinforced with time, harder to break and more 'normal' for the patient. It therefore becomes harder for them to see a need to change.

It can be useful (in order to gauge the patient's potential to benefit from this sort of cognitive work) to ask them to rate how much they believe a particular thought – either out of 10, or as a percentage. This can also offer a way of measuring treatment outcome; to see if, having challenged a negative thought, they believe it less.

For a patient to benefit from this sort of cognitive work, they need good insight, as they will first need to identify key fears and negative thoughts and understand when these occur. Anecdotally, a significant proportion of the older generation seem to benefit from a more behavioural approach, whereas younger patients seem more comfortable with the inclusion of talking-based therapy and cognitive work. However, Hynninen *et al.* (2010) completed a study of CBT (two hours each week, for seven weeks) with COPD patients who had anxiety and depression, and they found that age did not affect treatment response.

Encouraging positive thinking and coping thoughts

General positive thinking can be encouraged – for example, thoughts such as 'I will be OK' or 'I can cope'.

Likewise, breathlessness-targeted positive thoughts are helpful – for instance, 'My breathing will recover – it always has done before', 'I can cope with this' and 'I know that my breathing will gradually ease up'. If encouraging the patient to use these sorts of thoughts, you should always adapt them to use the patient's own language or turn of phrase.

A more individualised approach involves identifying unhelpful thoughts (as described in the previous section), improving the recognition of these thoughts when they come to mind, and challenging them. There are various ways to challenge them – for example, asking the patient what they would say to a friend who told them about the same fear or worry. This helps them gain some distance and a fresh perspective on their situation.

Another popular approach is to explore the evidence for and against the unhelpful thought/belief. For example, a patient who is anxious about going out of the house alone may have started to feel like this after experiencing a panic attack in a public place. They will have evidence for feeling anxious about going out alone, and it can be useful to acknowledge and validate these fears. However, you can then balance their fears by presenting evidence against the thought. For example, you could mention all the other times the person has been out alone and coped well, and remind them of the new strategies they can use to control breathlessness. This weighing up of the evidence provides a basis for the coping thought. If the coping thought is based on evidence, it is more believable and targets the root thinking patterns that trigger the adrenalin response.

Patients need to be reminded that negative patterns of thinking are easy to develop and often hard to break down. For a patient going out alone, an example of a coping thought might be 'I know this is anxiety because I haven't done this for ages. I can cope because I know I can stop and get my breath. I managed well when I did that walk with my daughter last week.'

When helpful, positive or coping thoughts have been identified, the patient can write them on statement cards. These cards can be kept in the patient's pocket, in their car, or anywhere in the house – preferably where they are easily visible in the rooms or places where they tend to have their breathlessness or panic episodes.

If using a coping thought that tackles negative, depressed thinking patterns, it can be useful to advise the patient to read the statement card several times a day. This is because they may not fully believe the coping thought initially but over time it will become more believable, especially if used in conjunction with behavioural interventions.

Behavioural interventions

Goal setting

You need to agree patient-centred goals that are meaningful to the patient in order to ensure engagement, and educate them about how to break a larger goal into smaller sections. Effective, skilled goal setting is vital for graded exposure treatment (in which the person gradually and increasingly faces an anxiety-provoking situation that they have been avoiding). It is very normal for realistic goal setting to develop over time, as the patient and health professional get to know what is possible. Remember that a patient may be able to do something within a supportive group setting but not necessarily when they are alone at home.

Increasing activity

Activity levels tend to be reduced in breathless patients because of their changing physical ability, but also because of reduced confidence, lack of interest and fear. If inactivity is due to fear of breathlessness, the following section will be useful. However, if inactivity is because of depression, treatment will be different. For depression, goal setting can focus on increasing activities that give (or used to give) a sense of pleasure (enjoyable activities) or mastery (being good at something). Goals should start small, as being able to achieve them is important in order to create a positive feedback loop that will bring the patient some satisfaction and sense of achievement.

Reducing avoidance behaviours

If unhelpful behaviours are to be changed and improved, they first need to be identified. It is not enough for a relative or health professional to identify problem behaviours such as avoiding exertion, or seeking reassurance by calling relatives often. The individual must recognise the behaviour as a problem and show some motivation to change. This is because it takes courage and is often uncomfortable to face breathlessness or anxiety when you have a history of fear. The relative or health professional can educate the patient about the long-term problems of avoidance (deconditioning, reduced confidence, increasing dependence, social isolation) and reassurance seeking (reduced independence, increased anxiety over time, and strain on supportive relationships). This basic education may need to be the starting point for treatment and assessing motivation to change.

The higher the anxiety and the longer the behaviour has been occurring, the smaller the goals must be. For example, a patient who has not been out of the house for several months but whose goal is to walk to the local shop alone, may start with walking a few steps away from the front door. They would then evaluate how they feel (perhaps rating their breathlessness and anxiety –

separately to increase insight – on a scale from 1 to 10). They would do this as often as possible until the score came down (e.g. below 5) and then the next step would be to walk to the nearest lamppost and back. The more frequently a patient works on a goal such as this, the faster their confidence and coping strategies will grow. Ideally they would try every day, and keep a diary of their scores and experiences. If a period as long as a week passes between each attempt, the positives of achieving the small goal are at risk of being taken over by the familiar negative thoughts. In addition, the long-term goal begins to feel unachievable.

Addressing the carer's thoughts and feelings about breathlessness can also be important in this process, as they may be inadvertently maintaining the avoidance. For example, they may make comments such as 'Do you think you should be doing that? What if you get too breathless and don't have anywhere to sit down?' Confidence building is a slow process for some people, but within a group setting (such as cardiac or pulmonary rehabilitation) the patient's self-efficacy in managing breathlessness often grows fast, as they observe others and feel safe to push themselves with health professionals nearby.

Distraction techniques

Distraction (moving attention away from the physical and psychological distress that the breathlessness may be causing) can be a simple and powerful technique. It allows time for the breathing to recover and prevents further anxious thoughts, which fuel physical symptoms. The distraction may be provided by a hobby. An activity that gives the patient the experience of 'flow' (losing track of time because they are so involved and enjoying it so much) is of immeasurable value.

In addition to hobbies, specific distraction techniques can be suggested. These can be many and varied, and may include:

- Recalling happy memories, perhaps with the aid of photos
- Word/number puzzle books
- Counting (e.g. back from 100 in 3s or 7s) or reciting a favourite poem (not aloud, as we would not want further energy or breath expended)
- Going out for a gentle walk (if able) or exercising, which will use up some of the extra energy that is being created as part of the adrenalin response

- Talking to a friend or relative (being careful not to take on their problems as well)
- Listening to the radio or some music or watching a favourite television programme.

Using several senses can be helpful so that a depth of distraction is achieved, and the mind and body are fully occupied with something else. In order to achieve this, the patient may choose to use more than one form of distraction simultaneously, e.g. listening to music and doing a word or number puzzle at the same time.

Social support and activity

It is not surprising that levels of social support have been positively linked with quality of life (Arne *et al.* 2011) and that high social support has been linked with low levels of anxiety and depression (Scherer *et al.* 2007). Encouraging a healthy amount of social engagement is not easy when a patient is breathless on exertion, low in confidence and possibly depressed. However, it is useful to ask about previous hobbies and interests. It may be necessary to build the patient's confidence to start a new activity but there are also a lot of social opportunities that are easily available in most communities and it is helpful for healthcare professionals to be familiar with them. For example, social contact can be gained through voluntary work, adult education courses, and day centres. Local connections with the British Heart Foundation or British Lung Foundation (Breathe Easy) groups (or equivalent charity-based services in other countries) and services in your area can all offer very useful resources. There may also be opportunities for patients who meet each other on a pulmonary or cardiac rehabilitation programme to continue regular contact and this should be encouraged. Some successfully support each other with exercise goals whilst others enjoy meeting and spending time with people who really understand what it is like to live with breathlessness.

Lifestyle balance and restructuring

Discussing the balance of a patient's life can empower them to recognise lifestyle factors that help or hinder their management of breathlessness. Lifestyle restructuring involves adapting activities to improve quality of life and management of their health condition. Sleep hygiene advice (e.g. having a relaxing routine before bed and reducing caffeine intake), assertiveness training and improving the balance of work, rest and leisure activities could be considered, alongside many of the stress management approaches discussed earlier in this chapter. Family therapy and relationship counselling may also be useful; relationship strain is quite common and understandable as partners, friends and family members adjust to the patient's deteriorating health and changes to their own roles and routines.

Relaxation techniques

The anxiety, frustration and panic spirals associated with breathlessness can cause rapid shallow breathing and muscle tension. Learning some simple relaxation techniques can help patients to control these emotions and breathe more easily.

There are a number of different relaxation techniques to choose from, including progressive muscle relaxation, autogenic relaxation, guided imagery and visualisation. Patients should choose the one that suits them best, and be encouraged to practise in a quiet, peaceful place at least once a day. The evidence for relaxation therapies is limited and is mostly based on studies of patients with COPD. Gift *et al.* (1992) and Renfroe (1988) showed that progressive muscle relaxation provided some relief from breathlessness in people with COPD. Another study of progressive muscle relaxation in chronic heart failure (CHF) found that, although psychological distress was reduced, there was little effect on breathlessness (Yu *et al.* 2007). Louie (2004) tested the effect of guided imagery on breathlessness in patients with COPD and found no significant difference in perceived breathlessness severity between the intervention (imagery group) and the control group.

Cued relaxation (in which the patient recognises the tension and then relaxes the tense muscle group) is useful to reduce the wasted energy expended when muscles are unnecessarily tense. It can be considered an aspect of fatigue management. For example, a patient could be encouraged to check their levels of tension every time they make a cup of tea or get in the car. The tension could be released by stretching the problem muscle area, or through the 'hold-tension-then-release' approach used in progressive muscular relaxation.

Reflection point

Helping a patient to manage anxiety can, in turn, lead to better control of breathlessness. Recognising anxiety-provoking situations and learning different coping strategies can transform the experience of breathlessness for some patients. Here are some useful tips to pass on to patients if you are unable to engage in more detailed psychological work:

- Recognise what triggers your anxiety
- Consider whether there are certain situations that make you feel more anxious
- Write down the kinds of things that worry or concern you
- Try to identify problems and solve them one at a time
- Mention how you are feeling to health professionals
- Learn a way of relaxing that works for you.

Mindfulness

Mindfulness is defined as paying attention in a particular way that is on purpose, in the present moment, and non-judgemental (Black 2011). Mindfulness courses are increasingly widely available and include specific techniques to improve the individual's ability to 'be in the moment' and not distracted by worries or fears. Techniques are sometimes taught as part of a wider treatment approach such as Acceptance and Commitment Therapy. Mindfulness-based stress reduction was mentioned in Chapter 5, (p. 81), when it was discussed in the context of CHF patients. Coventry and colleagues (2013) report from their systematic review and meta-analysis of the effect of complex interventions on depression and anxiety in COPD a non-statistically significant treatment effect following CBT interventions. They suggest that an acceptance response-based treatment involving mindfulness might be more appropriate for people with breathing-related anxiety. However, the evidence base for use of mindfulness techniques in physical health is small and has so far focused on other areas, such as pain management.

Motivation and overcoming barriers to change

Readiness to change

All healthcare professionals, especially those involved in rehabilitation and wanting to encourage self-management, can benefit greatly from an understanding of the stages of change, which underpin the motivational interviewing and counselling approach (Rollnick *et al.* 2010). For instance, there may be two patients with the same disease, the same severity and the same level of social support. However, one cannot recognise that there is a problem with his smoking or avoidance of exertion, and another is ready to make changes – but just needs a bit of guidance on what to do or how to do it. Using full counselling techniques would of course require more reading and training, but just being aware of the stages of change (pre-contemplation, contemplation, preparation, action and relapse) can help with:

- Assessing someone's suitability for rehabilitation (especially a group programme in which an individual can affect group dynamics)
- Understanding non-compliance and improving it
- Carrying out smoking cessation work
- Being more confident in assessing and understanding when the patient is not ready or not responding
- Assisting challenging patients – considering barriers to change.

Barriers to change

Considering a patient's 'barriers to change' can be a helpful way of getting some distance when viewing a non-compliant patient. This is important when frustration at the patient's lack of response to treatment, or the fact that they are taking little responsibility for managing their symptoms, can prove a challenge for the health professional involved. By considering barriers to change, the healthcare professional can adopt a stance of unconditional positive regard and a non-judgemental approach, which normalises ambivalence and recognises that motivation to change is affected by many different factors.

Some common barriers to change are:

- Untreated anxiety or depression
- Lack of support from a carer
- A higher-priority need (for example, if someone is about to be made homeless we cannot expect them to be able to consider breathing techniques)
- Stress

- Poor assertiveness skills
- Low confidence and self-efficacy
- Strongly held (unhelpful) health beliefs
- Unhelpful thought/behaviour spirals that have been reinforced over time.

Reflection point Reflection point Reflection point

When faced with a challenging patient, who may be expressing anger or being non-compliant, it is helpful to think of resistant behaviour as the problem, rather than perceiving the person as difficult. Consider the following. Maybe:

- They are not ready to change?
- They don't see that there is a problem?
- They don't believe they can change (low self-efficacy)?

Referring on

Be aware of the mental health services in your area and their criteria. There may be primary care mental health services or counselling available through the GP. For older people who are experiencing respiratory and cardiac problems, grief may also be affecting them, so consider bereavement services, and have helpline numbers available for other specific services (such as the Samaritans) to give patients who are expressing suicidal thoughts. Remember to access the voluntary sector as well as primary and secondary care services.

If you have an immediate concern about suicidal tendencies and level of risk, speak to the patient's GP and consider contacting your local community mental health team. Ask the patient directly about suicidal ideation and intent (NICE 2009). Patients often find it a relief to talk about suicidal thoughts freely but it can be difficult for the healthcare professional to know how to respond. Confidence in having these discussions grows with experience and you should request training from a local mental health provider to skill up your community team if necessary.

Always refer on (and liaise with other members of your team and the GP) if:

- You think the patient is at risk of harm to self/others
- You feel out of your depth
- You need advice/support.

General advice on managing stress related to breathlessness

It's always worth offering patients the following tips:

- Reduce your overall stress by lifestyle restructuring, relaxation and problem-solving
- Don't rush during activities or mobilising
- Communicate with friends and family about your limitations, e.g. having to walk more slowly
- Re-set expectations of how you will manage a task so that they are realistic – think about what you will be able to do (before starting the task)
- Accept that there will be good and bad days
- Know your limitations and set realistic goals for each day
- Understand the warning signs of a panic attack so that you can spot it early
- Use coping thoughts and distraction to counteract the panic
- Steer clear of the brown paper bag!! (This is sometimes used for panic but there is a risk of raising CO_2 which could be dangerous for some patients.)

Further information is available on the following websites:

www.BLF.org.uk – leaflets 'Dealing with Anxiety' and 'Dealing with Depression'

www.BHF.org.uk – leaflet 'Anxiety and Depression After a Heart Attack', 'Coping with Stress', HCP Factfile: Depression and Heart Disease

www.rcgp.org – patient leaflet 'Heart Disease and Mood' and HCP primary care guidance: Treating Depression in People with Coronary Heart Disease (January 2011)

www.rcpsych.ac.uk – improving physical and mental health, long-term conditions, links to useful leaflets for patients and HCPs

www.bemindful.co.uk – information on mindfulness

www.motivationalinterview.org – information on motivational interviewing

www.psychologytools.org – various resources, including links to Chris Williams' key articles on the five areas approach.

Reflection point

What do you think are the advantages and disadvantages of working with the breathless patient in their own home (as opposed to a hospital ward or clinic setting) when you are assessing or addressing psychological issues?

Summary

Many different psychological approaches can be used to understand and empower the breathless patient to cope with distressing breathlessness–emotion spirals. Careful assessment and understanding of the psychological impact of breathlessness is vital. Individualised psychoeducation, advice and coping strategies can then be worked on collaboratively with the patient, to build on other non-pharmacological strategies that are being used. The psychological treatment options can easily be overlooked within the medical model of practice, but patients will certainly benefit if psychological assessment and treatment can be embedded in specialist services.

References

Arne, M., Lundin, F., Boman, G., Janson, C., Janson, S. & Emtner, M. (2011). Factors associated with good self-rated health and quality of life in subjects with self-reported COPD. *International Journal of Chronic Obstructive Pulmonary Disease.* **6**, 511–19.

Black, D.S. (2011). A brief definition of mindfulness. Mindfulness Research Guide. Accessed from http://www.mindfulexperience.org

Bott, J., Blumenthal, S., Buxton, M. & Ellum, S. (2009). Guidelines for the physiotherapy management of the adult, medical, spontaneously breathing patient. *Thorax.* **64** (suppl1), i1–i51.

Coventry, P., Bower, P., Keyworth, C., Kenning, C., Knopp, J., Garrett, C., Hind, D., Malpass, A. & Dickens, C. (2013). The effect of complex interventions on depression and anxiety in chronic obstructive pulmonary disease: Systematic review and meta-analysis. PLoS ONE 8 (4): e60532. doi:10.1371/journal.pone.0060532.

Gift A.G., Moore T. & Soeken, K. (1992). Relaxation to reduce dyspnea and anxiety in COPD patients. *Nursing Research.* **41** (4), 242–6.

Gilbody., S., Richards., D. & Barkham, M. (2007). Diagnosing depression in primary care using self-completed instruments: UK validation of PHQ-9 and CORE-OM. *British Journal of General Practice.* **57** (541), 650–52.

Gysels, M. & Higginson, I. (2011). The lived experience of breathlessness and its implications for care: a qualitative comparison in cancer, COPD, heart failure and motor neuron disease. *BMC Palliative Care.* **10** (15).

Hall, A., Ferreira, P., Maher, G., Latimer, J. & Ferreira, M. (2010). The influence of the therapist–patient relationship on treatment outcome in physical rehabilitation: A systematic review. *Physical Therapy.* **90** (8), 1099–110.

Hynninen, M., Bjerke, N., Pallesen, S., Bakke, P. & Nordhus, I. (2010). A randomized controlled trial of cognitive behavioural therapy for anxiety and depression in COPD. *Respiratory Medicine.* **104**, 986–94.

Kübler-Ross, E. (1969). *On Death and Dying.* Routledge.

Kübler-Ross, E. (2005). *On Grief and Grieving: Finding the Meaning of Grief Through the Five Stages of Loss.* Simon & Schuster Ltd.

Lingen, C. (2007). Psychological distress in primary care patients with heart failure: a longitudinal study. *British Journal of General Practice.* **57** (543), 801–7.

Livermore, N., Sharpe, L. & McKenzie, D. (2010). Prevention of panic attacks and panic disorder in COPD. *European Respiratory Journal.* **35**, 557–63.

Louie, SW. (2004). The effects of guided imagery relaxation in people with COPD. *Occupational Therapy International.* **11** (3), 145–59.

Maurer, J., Rebbapragada, V., Borson, S., Goldstein, R., Kunik, M., Yohannes, A. & Hanania, N. (2008). Anxiety and depression in COPD: Current understanding, unanswered questions and research needs. *Chest.* **134**, 43S–56S.

National Institute for Clinical Excellence (NICE). (2009). Depression in adults with a chronic physical health problem. Treatment and management. http://www.nice.org.uk/nicemedia/pdf/CG91FullGuideline.pdf. Accessed online 30/04/2013.

National Institute for Clinical Excellence (NICE). (2011). Generalised anxiety disorder and panic disorder (with or without agoraphobia) in adults. Management in primary, secondary and community care. http://www.nice.org.uk/nicemedia/live/13314/52601/52601.pdf. Accessed online 30/04/2013.

Nici, L., Donner, C., Wouters, E., Zuwallack, R., Ambrosino, N., Bourbeau, J., Carone, M., Celli, B., Engelen, M., Fahy, B., Garvey, C., Goldstein, R. & Gosselink, R. (2006). American Thoracic Society/European Respiratory Society statement on pulmonary rehabilitation. *American Journal of Respiratory and Critical Care Medicine.* **173**, 1390–413.

Pierobon, A., Giardini, A., Callegari, S. & Majani, G. (2011). Psychological adjustment to a chronic illness: the contribution from cognitive behavioural treatment in a rehabilitation setting. *Giornale Italiano di Medicina del Lavoro ed Ergonomia.* **33** (1 Supplement A), A11–8.

Renfroe, K. (1988). Effect of progressive relaxation on dyspnea and state anxiety in patients with chronic obstructive pulmonary disease. *Heart Lung.* **17**, 408–13.

Rollnick, S., Butler, C., Kinnersley, P., Gregory, J. & Mash, B. (2010). Practice competent novice motivational interviewing. *British Medical Journal.* **340**, 1900.

Spitzer, R., Kroenke, K., Williams, J. & Löwe, B. (2006). A brief measure for assessing generalized anxiety disorder the GAD-7, *Archives of Internal Medicine.* **166** (10), 1092–7.

Scherer, M., Himmel, W., Stanske, H., Scherer, F., Koschack, J., Kochen, M. & Herrmann-Lingen, C. (2007). Psychological distress in primary care patients with heart failure: a longitudinal study. *British Journal of General Practice.* **57** (543), 801–7.

Williams, C. & Garland, A. (2002). A cognitive-behavioural therapy assessment model for use in everyday clinical practice. *Advances in Psychiatric Treatment.* **8**, 172–9.

Yohannes, A.M., Willgoss, T.G., Baldwin, R.C. & Connolly, M.J. (2010). Depression and anxiety in chronic heart failure and chronic obstructive pulmonary disease: prevalence, relevance, clinical implications and management principles. *International Journal of Geriatric Psychiatry.* **25** (12), 1209–21.

Yu, D.S.F., Lee, D.T.F. & Woo, J. (2007). Effect of relaxation on psychologic distress and symptom status in older Chinese patients with heart failure. *Journal of Psychosomatic Research.* **62**, 5427–437.

10

Pharmacological management of breathlessness

Patrick White

The opening chapter of this book highlighted the need for accurate diagnosis of breathlessness as a presenting symptom in primary care and for the underlying cause to be treated appropriately. Only when breathlessness persists, despite our best efforts to control its cause, should thought be given to interventions to relieve it as a symptom. The symptomatic treatment of breathlessness tends to be a late intervention in the disease that is causing the breathlessness. When symptomatic treatment of breathlessness is needed, drugs are usually the second line of treatment – after physical measures have been tried. The clinician should first ask if adequate consideration has been given to the non-pharmacological measures described earlier in this book and particularly in Chapters 8 and 9. In this sense, pharmacological treatment of the symptom of breathlessness is a last resort. It does not tackle the underlying cause, it has no impact on the course of the disease, and it may bring about side effects that complicate the overall management of the patient.

The symptomatic treatment of breathlessness with drugs is an area that has been under-researched and poorly resourced. Patients with intractable breathlessness have been inappropriately or under-treated because of widespread ignorance about which interventions are effective and how they should be used. Too often, breathless patients have been given oxygen when it was ineffective in relieving their symptoms, or they have been given opiates in inappropriate doses.

In this chapter, I will describe the context in which breathlessness should be managed in the community and the size of the problem. I will suggest an approach to the identification and structured care of breathless patients, and will briefly describe the drugs (including oxygen) used in the symptomatic relief of breathlessness in the community. The specific management of the commoner causes of breathlessness is dealt with elsewhere in this book (see Chapters 3–6), and the symptomatic treatment of breathlessness in advanced disease at the end of life is further described in Chapter 11.

The context of breathlessness management in the community

Breathlessness is a highly subjective symptom, the perception of which arises from combinations of hypoxia, hypercapnia, acidosis, muscle fatigue, changes in muscle proprioception, changes in neural regulation, bronchial narrowing, lung restriction, dynamic hyperinflation and tachycardia. The particular contribution of each of these influences varies between patients. Confirming their severity with physiological measurement is fraught with difficulty because breathlessness is subjective, and often has to be described using words rather than physiological measurements. The perception of breathlessness is further complicated by its long-term nature, and by the degree to which the patient has become accustomed to it. For example, a cancer patient approaching the end of life may find the sudden onset of breathlessness much harder to tolerate than a patient with a chronic lung or heart condition (who has had progressive breathlessness for ten years) or a patient with heart failure (who has had progressive breathlessness for one or two years).

The challenge posed by breathlessness in a community setting should be assessed in terms of respiratory rate, heart rate and hypoxia. Having identified the underlying cause, a decision can be made on the danger represented by the breathlessness and the urgency of intervention. From that point on, the breathlessness may be the main impetus for further presentation of the patient. It then becomes the spur to assessment and disease-specific treatments, which may be physical, psychological or pharmacological.

Prolonged exposure to breathlessness may lead to response shift – a resetting of perception of the symptom and the internal response to it

(Schwartz & Sprangers 1999). Thus the patient may undergo a recalibration of the importance and perceived severity of their breathlessness. Individuals with very severe impairment over long periods may therefore seem less distressed than patients with apparently less severe impairment that has come on acutely.

These differences in context are important in determining when and how drugs should be used to control the symptom of breathlessness (rather than control the disease). Patients with advanced chronic diseases, who have lived with breathlessness for several years, demand a different approach from those whose death from cancer is imminent and in whom the symptom of breathlessness is recent. Physical strategies, including rehabilitation programmes that counteract the de-conditioning effect of chronic illness, can improve exercise capacity, reduce breathlessness, and improve the quality of life of patients with chronic disease. However, they are inappropriate for patients whose health and capacity are deteriorating rapidly. These are the patients whose breathlessness may be transformed by drugs.

The decision to prescribe drugs to control breathlessness may seem least challenging in advanced cancer, when the patient's life expectancy is dramatically reduced (Booth, Moosavi & Higginson 2008). In patients with breathlessness due to chronic disease, the clinician must ensure that the disease itself is optimally managed, and should consider physical measures to control the breathlessness before resorting to drug treatment of the symptom.

In chronic disease, ineffective or sub-optimal treatment of the underlying disease is easy to miss. Too often, for example, inappropriate inhalers are prescribed for patients with COPD who are unable to use them. Pressurised metered dose inhalers are the most widely prescribed and the cheapest devices for the delivery of drugs in COPD. They are also the most difficult to use, and may therefore account for commonly missed causes of under-treatment of these diseases. In chronic heart failure, many patients miss out on the life-extending benefits of careful calibration of angiotensin-converting enzyme inhibitors with beta-blockers, spironolactone, and loop diuretics to improve cardiac efficiency, and reduce breathlessness and peripheral oedema. Drug treatments for the symptomatic control of breathlessness should not be introduced in such patients before the underlying disease is optimally treated.

Case study 10.1

PJ, a 68-year-old retired factory manager, had COPD. He had been prescribed salbutamol 100mcg/dose (to be used 2–4 puffs four-hourly if needed in a pMDI), combined salmeterol and fluticasone (25/250) pMDI, and tiotropium 30mg powder capsules for inhalation. Having attended monthly for three months, he continued to complain of breathlessness on minimal exertion. His FEV_1 was 88L/min, 25% of the FEV_1 expected for his age and height. On this attendance, his inhaler technique was tested again. He had great difficulty synchronising the inhalation with his breathing, with the result that much of the inhaled gas slipped out the corner of his mouth and down his nose. His pMDIs were changed to powder inhalers. After four weeks his FEV_1 had risen to 170L/min, demonstrating a partially reversible component to his airway obstruction (mixed asthma and COPD) and offering the possibility of reduced exacerbations of his COPD.

By the time it has been decided to introduce drugs to improve the symptomatic control of breathlessness, the clinician should be confident that every opportunity has been taken to control the underlying disease, that all physical and psychological measures have been considered, and that the patient's distress demands further intervention in its own right.

Breathless patients make up a significant proportion of the workload in the community or primary care setting but the treatment they require is largely aimed at managing the disease. Patients that mainly require symptom control interventions are usually in the advanced stages of their disease. An average practice of 6500 patients with four GPs and one or two practice nurses is likely to have only a few patients with intractable breathlessness due to COPD (White *et al.* 2011). The number with severe breathlessness due to cancer is harder to pinpoint. Many of these patients are housebound and only present to their GP when they become acutely ill. We know that more than 30% of people who die of COPD in the UK had not been seen by their GP or specialist doctor in the three months before their deaths. Some patients may be in contact with nurse specialist outreach teams who are likely to provide advice regarding non-pharmacological management of breathlessness.

Identifying and managing breathless patients in the community

Chapter 1 described the systematic approaches to patient care that can radically improve the identification and management of breathless patients with advanced disease. The numbers of patients requiring pure symptomatic assessment of breathlessness each year are likely to be small – of the order of 2–3 per GP or 8–10 per average practice.

The vast majority of breathless patients in the community are managed using disease-specific treatments. There is good evidence that management of these patients can be variable. Before patients are considered for breathlessness symptom management, their disease-specific management should be optimal. Many of the physical and non-pharmacological interventions used in breathless patients, and described in detail earlier in this chapter, should be prescribed as part of the disease-specific management cycle. Cardiac and pulmonary rehabilitation are very effective in moderate disease, significantly improving breathlessness, exercise capacity and quality of life. Some patients are extremely sensitive to breathlessness, which they find emotionally overwhelming and which can lead to crippling anxiety. Training in breathing management and anxiety control may be transformative in such patients, long before the strategies for disease management have been exhausted.

Breathless patients should also be assessed for hypoxia. There are three reasons for this. The first is to identify patients who are so hypoxic that they would gain symptomatic benefit from diurnal oxygen. The second is to identify patients who desaturate on exercise and require ambulatory oxygen to enable them to exercise safely. The third reason is to identify COPD patients who may be suffering from chronic hypoxia, in whom pulmonary hypertension should be prevented.

Breathless patients who require symptom control with drugs usually have advanced disease. They comprise a small group of patients in a community setting, and most general practitioners and community-based nurses will have limited experience of their management. In the past, such patients were only given disease-specific treatments or were given oxygen in the hope of relieving the breathlessness. We now know that opiates can significantly improve the daily experience of these patients, and oxygen is only rarely helpful. Clinicians in a community setting should therefore seek the help of community palliative care teams, specialist breathlessness clinics, or respiratory or cardiac specialists with an interest in advanced disease, when treating breathless patients who need symptom control in advanced disease.

Oxygen

Oxygen is an unreliable treatment for breathless patients if its use is not tied to objective evidence of hypoxaemia (O'Driscoll, Howard & Davison 2011). It should be remembered that oxygen is a treatment for hypoxaemia, not breathlessness. In patients who are acutely ill and breathless, oxygen saturation should be checked by pulse oximetry. In chronically ill breathless patients, hypoxaemia can be screened with pulse oximetry and for those whose oxygen saturation (SpO_2) is less than 92% arterial blood gases should be checked. This advice also applies to palliative care patients who are approaching the end of life, with cancer or chronic respiratory or cardiac disease, although treatment should not be delayed if it is impractical to assess arterial blood gases. Pulse oximetry should be available to all community clinicians who are assessing and treating breathlessness. It is particularly useful in assessing breathless patients who are approaching the end of life because oxygen can be ordered and delivered urgently if needed for those who are hypoxaemic. However, for most patients approaching end of life, pulse oximetry will demonstrate that they are not hypoxaemic and that oxygen is therefore not indicated.

The majority of patients for whom home oxygen should be prescribed have COPD. In these patients, the goal of long-term oxygen therapy (LTOT) is to reduce hypoxia in the alveolar capillaries in order to prevent pulmonary hypertension. Pulmonary hypertension is the cause of right heart failure in chronically hypoxaemic COPD patients. Its prevention is one of the few interventions that can improve life expectancy in COPD, the others being smoking cessation and drugs that reduce the frequency of disease exacerbations. Oxygen is also used to treat hypoxaemia in other respiratory diseases and for hypoxaemic patients with cardiac or neurological diseases. A small proportion of COPD patients with severe lung disease suffer from desaturation of oxygen on exercise, with resultant reduced exercise capacity due to breathlessness. Such patients will benefit from ambulatory oxygen therapy during exercise if their oxygen saturation falls by more than 4% to an SpO_2 level of less than 90%.

Many patients report relief of breathlessness after administration of oxygen despite the absence of hypoxia. However, this is probably related to the soothing effect of the gas flowing over the face (similar to the effect of a hand-held fan) and may be unrelated to the actual delivery of oxygen.

Opiates

The most widely used drug for the symptomatic control of breathlessness is morphine and this is also the drug with the best evidence base. Morphine is thought to act by altering the ventilator response to carbon dioxide, hypoxia and inspiratory flow resistive loading, and by reducing the consumption of oxygen at rest and during exercise. Mahler and colleagues demonstrated the production of endogenous opiates during exercise in an experiment with COPD patients (Mahler *et al.* 2009). When they administered naloxone to block the effect of the endogenous opiates, breathlessness was made worse. Morphine can be used by breathless patients in their homes but its prescription should be supervised by a clinician experienced in using it for the breathlessness control. This will usually require the involvement of a palliative specialist physician or nurse, or a respiratory or cardiac physician, to support the community or primary care clinician.

Morphine has been shown to be effective in reducing breathlessness by oral and parenteral administration in a number of randomised controlled trials (Johnson, Abernethy & Currow 2012). However, there is no evidence that it is effective in nebulised form. Currow and colleagues have shown that morphine is effective at daily doses of 10mg, and its benefit is sustained at that dosage for up to three months (Currow *et al.* 2011). Doses should be increased in 25% increments until symptoms are relieved. At these levels, there is no evidence of risk of respiratory depression. Familiarity with the treatment of breathlessness with opiates is important because the principles of treatment are different from those that govern pain management. Of particular importance is the careful stepping up of dosages in modest stages and the expectation of symptom relief at relatively low levels of drug dosage. There is limited evidence to support the use of other opiates but it is thought that the effect of morphine is a class effect and not specific to the molecule itself. Other opiate drugs that have been used in the symptomatic treatment of breathlessness are hydromorphone and nebulised fentanyl.

Case study 10.2

JA, a 74-year-old retired taxi driver with ischaemic heart disease, had been suffering from heart failure for the previous five years. He had progressive breathlessness despite careful optimising of his drugs, which included ramipril 10mg, bisoprolol 5mg and spironolactone 50mg, and despite regular exercise after undertaking cardiac rehabilitation. He used frusemide 40mg daily when his ankle swelling and breathlessness got worse and his weight rose. For at least three months, he was distressed by breathlessness on minimal exertion and was increasingly exhausted. He was seen by his specialist heart failure nurse, together with a specialist palliative care physician, and started on morphine sulphate liquid, 10mg/5ml, 1.25ml six-hourly. There was a significant improvement in his breathlessness, he was sleeping less fitfully, and he was noticeably less fatigued and anxious. His morphine was changed to morphine sulphate, modified release tablets, 5mg twice daily, and after two months was increased to 10mg twice daily. For the next two months, he remained stable and reported being relatively comfortable, albeit breathless on minimal exertion.

Other drugs

Benzodiazepines have been used in the treatment of dyspnoea for many years, with little evidence of their effectiveness. This is certainly true of diazepam and chlordiazepoxide. Benzodiazepines are administered because of the presence of anxiety and panic associated with breathlessness. However, a systematic review found no benefit from these drugs, compared to placebo, for the management of breathlessness (Simon *et al.* 2010). Recently, oral midazolam was compared with oral morphine in a randomised controlled trial, which involved rapid titration of the two drugs against symptoms increasing in 25% doses (Navigante, Castro & Cerchiette 2010). The starting dose for morphine was 3mg and that for midazolam was 2mg. Midazolam was as effective as morphine in relieving severe breathlessness. Side effects (mainly mild somnolence) were similar in both groups. Midazolam should only be prescribed in these circumstances by a clinician with specialist support.

One promising therapy is mirtazapine. Mirtazapine is a commonly used antidepressant with good evidence supporting its use in major depressive disorders associated with anxiety (Watanabe *et al.* 2008). It is available in tablet, oro-dispersible and liquid formations and has a simple dosing and titration regime (Watanabe *et al.* 2008). Its mechanisms of action for breathlessness are likely to involve modulation of the respiratory rhythm and on processing of breathlessness perception in the brain cortex (see Chapter 2) and anxiety reduction. Further research into the potential benefits of mirtazapine for the control of breathlessness would be warranted.

A study of 12 stable patients with COPD randomised to receive 50mcg nebulised fentanyl or placebo prior to a constant work rate cycle exercise test showed increased exercise endurance in the fentanyl group. There was no difference in breathlessness intensity or unpleasantness, but the rate of rise of breathlessness intensity was slower in the fentanyl group. This finding warrants further exploration, and also highlights the issue that exercise endurance in the ambulant person may be the more important factor, rather than breathlessness intensity (Jensen *et al.* 2011).

Nebulised furosemide has been used in the symptomatic treatment of breathlessness because of its observed effect in relieving cough. Furosemide is a commonly prescribed loop diuretic. When inhaled as a mist, it has a variety of actions on lung parenchyma that inhibit cough and protect against bronchoconstrictor stimuli (Booth, Moosavi & Higginson 2008). Studies of experimental breathlessness in healthy subjects indicate that breathlessness relief might be mediated by modulation of sensory afferent signals from irritant or stretch receptors (see Chapter 2) (Booth, Moosavi & Higginson 2008, Ventresca *et al.* 1990). A number of case reports and uncontrolled trials of inhaled furosemide have indicated that it might relieve breathlessness in terminal cancer patients (Shimoyama & Shimoyama 2002) but no clinical trials exist. At present, its use should be considered experimental.

Summary

Managing the symptom of breathlessness with drugs should always be the treatment of last resort, after optimal treatment of the underlying disease and careful use of physical and supportive treatments. Use of oxygen should be restricted to treatment of hypoxaemia, except in advanced or terminal disease where oxygen saturation cannot be measured. Oral drug treatment with morphine and benzodiazepines has a growing evidence base. The use of these drugs is likely to become more widespread in advanced respiratory and cardiac disease, as we increase our understanding of dosage, tolerance, and side effects in these patients. The dangers associated with these drugs in the treatment of breathlessness probably lie in using them at doses more suitable for chronic pain, and in titrating them upwards at inappropriate rates.

References

Booth, S., Moosavi, S.H. & Higginson, I.J. The etiology and management of intractable breathlessness in patients with advanced cancer: a systematic review of pharmacological therapy. (2008). *Nature Clinical Practice Oncology.* **5** (2), 90–100.

Currow, D.C., McDonald, C., Oaten, S., Kenny, B., Allcroft, P. & Frith, P. (2011). Once-daily opioids for chronic dyspnea: a dose increment and pharmacovigilance study. *Journal of Pain and Symptom Management.* **42** (3), 388–99.

Jensen, D., Alsuhail, A., Viola, R., Dudgeon, D.J., Webb, K.A., O'Donnell, D.E. (2011). Inhaled fentanyl citrate improves exercise endurance during high-intensity constant work rate cycle exercise in chronic obstructive pulmonary disease. *Journal of Pain and Symptom Management.* **43**, vol 4, pp. 706 - 719.

Johnson, M.J., Abernethy, A.P & Currow, D.C. Gaps in the evidence base of opioids for refractory breathlessness. A future work plan? (2012). *Journal of Pain and Symptom Management.* **26**.

Mahler, D.A., Murray, J.A., Waterman, L.A., Ward, J., Kraemer, W.J. & Zhang, X. (2009). Endogenous opioids modify dyspnoea during treadmill exercise in patients with COPD. *European Respiratory Journal.* **33** (4), 771–7.

Navigante, A.H., Castro, M.A. & Cerchietti, L.C. (2010). Morphine versus midazolam as upfront therapy to control dyspnea perception in cancer patients while its underlying cause is sought or treated. *Journal of Pain and Symptom Management.* **39** (5), 820–30.

O'Driscoll, B.R., Howard, L.S. & Davison, A.G. (2011). Emergency oxygen use in adult patients: concise guidance. *Clinical Medicine.* **11** (4), 372–5.

Schwartz, C.E. & Sprangers, M.A. (1999). Methodological approaches for assessing response shift in longitudinal health-related quality-of-life research. *Social Science Medicine.* **48** (11), 1531–48.

Shimoyama, N. & Shimoyama, M. (2002). Nebulized furosemide as a novel treatment for dyspnea in terminal cancer patients. *Journal of Pain Symptom Management.* **23**, 73–6.

Simon, S.T., Higginson, I.J., Booth, S., Harding, R. & Bausewein, C. (2010). Benzodiazepines for the relief of breathlessness in advanced malignant and non-malignant diseases in adults. Cochrane Database Syst Rev. 20(1):CD007354. doi: 10.1002/14651858.CD007354.pub2.

Ventresca, P.G., Nichol, G.M., Barnes, P.J. & Chung, K.F. (1990). Inhaled furosemide inhibits cough induced by low chloride content solutions but not by capsaicin. *American Review of Respiratory Disease.* **142**, 143–6.

Watanabe, N., Omori, I.M., Nakagawa, A., Cipriani, A., Barbui, C., McGuire, H., Churchill, R. & Furukawa, T.A.; Multiple Meta-Analyses of New Generation Antidepressants (MANGA) Study Group. (2008). Mirtazapine versus other antidepressants in the acute-phase treatment of adults with major depression: systematic review and meta-analysis. *The Journal of Clinical Psychiatry.* **69** (9), 1404–15.

White, P., White, S., Edmonds, P., Gysels, M., Moxham, J. & Seed, P. (2011). Palliative care or end-of-life care in advanced chronic obstructive pulmonary disease: A prospective community survey. *British Journal of General Practice.* **61** (587), 362–70.

11

End-of-life breathlessness management at home

Sara Booth and Julie Burkin

This chapter is concerned with caring for someone at home at the end of life, when breathlessness is the major symptom. It mainly focuses on care given by allied health professionals (AHPs) but considers all the care that needs to be given by the multidisciplinary team. It is based on the available evidence in the literature, but also on 'best practice', as this is not an area where there has been much research. Having the confidence and expertise to deviate from an algorithm to treat an individual and a family in a tailor-made way is very important; seniority, confidence, training and excellent teamwork are vital.

When a person is breathless and likely to die in the next few days, weeks or even months, it is essential that preparations are made for the end of life as early in the disease course as possible. This is of course desirable for most end-of-life care but, since breathless patients have a much higher chance of being admitted to hospital to die and/or of needing sedation, it is even more critical for them. If a patient wants to stay at home for the final stages, it is essential that plans are put in place as soon as this has been discussed.

Uncontrolled breathlessness is a terrifying symptom for both sufferers and onlookers, particularly close family members. It has increasingly been realised that breathlessness management is most effective if it is started when breathlessness is predicted rather than after it has started. In other words, for any patient with advanced cardio-respiratory disease, particularly cancer affecting the thorax, COPD or interstitial lung disease (ILD), many of the most effective treatments are non-pharmacological and require the patient to change long-standing habits. It has also been recognised that the carer, being a key person in breathlessness management, needs support and help and that breathlessness will be better controlled when this happens (Booth *et al.* 2003, Booth *et al.* 2011). It is also critical to remember that carers have health and psychological needs of their own.

Principles of best practice in end-of-life breathlessness management

The following principles are based on best practice, to help make it more likely that the 'desired death' will be achieved at home:

1 Achieve the best symptom control as soon as possible
2 Understand and support carers' needs
3 Arrange advanced care planning
4 Ensure that all services likely to be needed are alerted and preferably know the patient.

1 Achieve the best symptom control as soon as possible

A patient with uncontrolled breathlessness, who has no idea how to manage a breathlessness attack and whose relatives feel similarly unskilled, is unlikely to be able to stay at home to die, however strongly they may initially wish to do this. Even if they can live with the idea of having uncontrolled breathlessness at home, their partner or other family members almost certainly won't be able to tolerate it. Any clinicians (such as paramedics) who are visiting out of hours, and come across someone with uncontrolled breathlessness, will feel that they must immediately admit that person to hospital.

Clinicians giving end-of-life care to people at home will not have any control over the stage at which patients are referred to them. However, if they are working in a particular area and routinely find that patients are referred to them too late, they need to address this with clinicians and managers, perhaps by setting up an advanced multidisciplinary team (MDT).

If you are the clinician to whom someone living at home (with advanced disease and uncontrolled breathlessness) has been referred, your first priority must be to work as hard as possible to achieve symptom control. This is likely to mean intensive work to get enough caring agencies on board to provide the range of services that this patient needs (Spathis & Booth 2008, Spathis *et al.* 2011). Without physical, hands-on and expert symptom control, a patient with advanced disease and breathlessness will not be able to stay at home. If a clinician has to introduce extra help in the home as an emergency at the very end of life, this is much more difficult for the family to accept because there is little time for them to build up any rapport and therefore have confidence in the new carer. Ideally, terminal patients with breathlessness will be assessed months or weeks (not days) before death and the family will become familiar with the carers early on. Sadly, as funding is restricted, hands-on care will often only be introduced when the patient needs specific tasks done. However, hospice services can often come in earlier in order to build up a relationship with the patient and their family.

Reflection point

Getting control of breathlessness, in order to reduce suffering and gain the confidence of the patient and the family, is the first priority when caring for the breathless patient at home.

If the patient accepts the idea of being admitted to a hospice but not an acute hospital at the end of life, it is essential that they are introduced to the hospice early on, perhaps by visiting the hospice day centre or by having regular contact with AHPs from Hospice at Home. It may even be possible for them to have a 'symptom control admission' well before death and to be discharged back home with support from the hospice. This will increase the likelihood of the patient being able to die at home. If it is agreed that hospice care is appropriate for a patient with non-malignant disease (such as COPD, CHF, ILD or PH) who is still under the care of respiratory physicians, it should be made clear and agreed in writing, during normal working hours, what contingencies would take the person into the hospice as an emergency, or what would need to be assessed in the acute hospital with early transfer to the hospice. One of the eventualities is that a patient with, for example, COPD is seen by an out-of-hours doctor or paramedic who has not met them before and has no notes about them. This staff member admits the patient to the hospital because they are concerned about the possibility of an acute exacerbation. The patient then dies in hospital, without ever getting back home or to the hospice. This is where a prior discussion (agreeing and recording preferred priorities of care) is particularly useful, as it can ensure that the patient's wishes are carried out. When discussed, documented and shared with the wider clinical team in a timely and appropriate manner, advanced care planning helps to ensure that the patient can exercise a degree of control and choice over their care at the end of their lives.

Reflection point

If you have a discussion about priorities for care (for example, if the patient prefers to be admitted to a hospice rather than an acute ward if they have a further exacerbation), it is essential that this decision is:

- Agreed with other clinicians
- Communicated widely after being recorded so that, for instance, the ambulance service is not put in an impossible position and forced to admit the patient to hospital.

2 Understand and support carers' needs

The majority of carers of patients with advanced disease and breathlessness are likely to be elderly, although this is not always the case. Anyone caring for someone who is seriously ill is subject to huge physical and psychological demands. After months or even years of caring for a very sick patient at home, they are likely to be both mentally and physically exhausted, particularly if there has been no assessment or consideration of their emotional and physical needs. Carers also often express sadness at the 'loss' of the routine of life as it was, prior to the patient becoming unwell. Very often they will have co-morbidities of their own. They may have neglected their own health or lost contact with other friends and family. They may have had no respite from caring for their relative. Caring can have detrimental effects on an individual's health, even if they were fit before they took on the role. When the breathlessness gets worse towards the end of life, as it commonly will, they may therefore be unable to call on inner resources to enable them to look after the person at home.

Carers' needs should therefore be addressed as early as patients' needs, and adequate help and respite should be offered (perhaps, for example, in the form of the patient attending the hospice day centre). In addition, the carer needs to know where they can go for help; and when they ask for help, they should get it quickly and easily. They also need a chance to discuss their own fears and concerns about the illness and the symptom of breathlessness. It is not at all unusual (in fact it is the norm) for wives, husbands, brothers, sisters, sons or daughters (or any other combination of carer and patient) to cope very differently with the same situation. While one will want to talk at some length about what is happening, another will find it more helpful to deny or 'switch off', perhaps preferring to focus only on dealing with practical issues.

Reflection point Reflection point Reflection point

If you do not tend to the carer's needs, you will not be able to keep a sick patient with breathlessness at home. At some point the carer will become unwell (mentally or physically or both) if their needs are not attended to.

3 Arrange advanced care planning

Advanced care planning involves:

- Finding out what the patient wants for their end-of-life care
- Finding out what the carer needs to help the patient achieve their desired end-of-life care
- Putting in place the services that will enable this to happen
- Ensuring that the plans are written down and communicated to all the agencies caring for the patient.

The process of advanced care planning is particularly helpful when looking towards the future and it gives individuals an opportunity to think about, talk about and write down their priorities for care. This could mean agreeing that the patient may come into the hospice (rather than hospital) in emergencies, or that they will stay at home whatever happens, or that they will have a Hospice at Home arrangement. It may also mean making sure that primary care services (whether routine, 'out of hours' or ambulance services) know that they must not bring that patient into hospital if they are called, unless it is completely unavoidable. These plans are much more likely to be adhered to if they are made early so that the necessary caring services can be put in place. Early planning also means that these issues can be raised with patients and families sensitively, under the 'hope for the best, but plan for the worst' approach, ensuring that patients get the treatment they really want as they get less well.

Reflection point Reflection point Reflection point

If the subject of end-of-life planning is approached insensitively, as if it were another routine enquiry, it can be extremely distressing for the patient and their family. You are likely to lose their confidence and the subject may never be broached again.

Find out first if anyone else has discussed it with the patient and then take your cue from the patient about how to talk about this difficult issue. If you are uncertain, ask for help *early* – for example, from your local specialist palliative care service.

4 Ensure that all services likely to be needed are alerted and preferably know the patient

It may be unavoidable for a patient to see a service at the end of life with whom they are completely unfamiliar. However, end-of-life care is more likely to be effective when patients are familiar with the caring services and have started to make contact with them when they are relatively well, rather than meeting them for the first time in the last days of life. Extra services will probably be needed to help the patient stay at home, and the patient needs to meet the people providing those services early on, when they do not need them every day. The services that are going to help the patient achieve symptom control rapidly are the ones they need to meet first. There is nothing worse for patients and family than having crowds of different clinical services entering the house (in a disruptive and time-consuming way), achieving nothing and merely taking down the same details and history as the previous service. For someone with breathlessness, a palliative care service (particularly a breathlessness service) should be the earliest referral outside primary care. Such services may be based in hospices or hospitals. As with any other stage of care, effective and efficient communication is the key to ensuring that the patients' wishes are being adhered to. Accurate documentation is also vital, particularly when a number of services are involved.

Management of the symptom of breathlessness

Symptom management is described in detail elsewhere but the key areas in symptom control are outlined here. As patients reach the end of life, pharmacological treatment becomes more important than non-pharmacological treatments. However, pharmacological treatment alone will not be enough to manage the whole situation. The key treatments for the symptom itself (rather than the fear it generates) are pharmacological. The breathless patient with advanced disease is very likely to be taking oral opioids to help reduce the impact of the symptom. However, even patients at the end of life may not have been started on these useful medicines. If you find someone with uncontrolled breathlessness, it is therefore important to get them assessed for the possibility of introducing opioids and sometimes benzodiazepines or other oral anxiolytic drugs. These drugs can be started either by the specialist breathlessness service or by the family doctor or respiratory physician. Alerting these allied health professionals (AHPs) to the possibility that the patient may need these drugs could be an important part of your role. When the patient is dying, opioids and benzodiazepines can be given subcutaneously (see Table 11.1, page 176) (Booth 2009). One of your most important roles when caring for the patient at the end of life is to reassure them about the use of drugs. Drug therapy can make an important, positive difference and drugs do not have to be used at sedative doses.

Non-pharmacological treatments for breathlessness are outlined in Chapter 8. However, at the end of life the most important psychological support you can offer patients is simply to be competent and available, clearly listening to their concerns and acting on them. If patients feel isolated, their anxiety and distress are likely to spiral out of control.

Psychological support

The mind and body are inextricably linked, and fear, terror and anxiety can clearly precipitate or exacerbate episodes of breathlessness. At this stage, it will probably be too difficult for patients to start learning non-pharmacological anxiety reduction techniques, such as cognitive behavioural therapy (CBT) in its most rigorous form. However, they can be supported in using cognitive approaches that they have already learned. At the very end of life, the following psychological approaches may be useful:

- **Advice and education**: For example, it can be very useful to remind the patient that, although it is frightening and unpleasant, breathlessness is not in itself harmful and will reduce on its own. The carer can also be supported in reminding the patient of this.
- **Breathing retraining**: Helping patients to manage their breathing pattern, and use the fan in a 'breathe-as-you-go' way (see http://www.cuh.org.uk/breathlessness) can be very supportive. Remember to refer patients to resources, such as websites, which can continue education in the home even when the clinician is not there.
- **Supported mindfulness/self-hypnosis or visualisation**: The clinician can help the patient to get into 'a safe or special place' and mentally disassociate from the fear and anxiety around them.

If the patient (or carer) is able to acquire any of these strategies, they can be used at any time to reduce dependency and promote self-efficacy. Again, they are most effective if taught by a clinician early on in a day therapy centre, outpatients department or in the home, before being needed at the end of life.

Reflection point Reflection point Reflection point

Although a very sick patient cannot exercise, helping them to be as mentally and physically active as possible can make an important difference to their own and their carers' quality of life. If someone can transfer from bed to chair, or commode, life will be so much easier at home.

Equipment

Extra equipment can be very helpful as the patient becomes weaker. It is vital to undertake a thorough assessment of the patient, their abilities, the carer and the environment in order to ensure accurate equipment prescription. The items of equipment that are likely to be most useful include:

- **Walking aids**: These enable the patient to continue to be mobile on their own for as long as possible. This will not only help the patient to feel more in control and less dependent but can also spare the relative or carer from having to do hundreds of small, exhausting and irritating errands.
- **Wheelchairs**: These can be helpful in terms of enabling the patient to continue with outdoor activities with the family and they are also a very useful way of encouraging the patient to pace themselves – for example, using a wheelchair to do the boring part of an outing (e.g. car park to venue) and then walking for a while once there, using the chair for further support when necessary.
- **A monkey pole**: This may enable a weakened patient to pull themselves up in bed without help, increasing independence. However, care needs to be taken when prescribing this piece of equipment, as it can place considerable strain on the muscles and joints of the upper body, which may exacerbate pain issues.
- **Bedside rails or a bed lever**: These may enable a patient to roll themselves on to one side, to assist with personal hygiene or positioning. Bed levers can also assist with transfers in and out of bed.
- **Slide sheets**: These can be very useful in assisting with positioning in bed, such as manoeuvring patients up and down the bed or rolling on to their side. They are helpful in minimising the effort required by the patient.
- **A slide board**: This can help patients and relatives manoeuvre from bed to chair when the person is unable to fully weight-bear. Note that this piece of equipment does rely on the person having sufficient balance and upper body strength to use safely.
- **A hoist**: This is often considered essential when a patient is bed bound, and most services will now insist on a hoist being in the house if they are to do any significant moving and handling. However, it may be worth considering whether the person does actually need to be moved from bed or whether they can be managed entirely in bed if this is more comfortable for them.
- **Pressure mattresses**: These are available to mitigate the risk of pressure areas and pressure sores in these high-risk patients, to increase comfort and to minimise the need for turning, which patients often find distressing, particularly in the very last days or hours of life.
- **A hospital bed**: This may be required toward the end of life. However, there is often at least a 48-hour delay before it arrives so it is important to

anticipate in good time that a patient is going to be bed-bound and will need nursing from both sides. It is also important to identify early on a place where the bed can go and preferably organise a room downstairs where the patient can be nursed. This may also increase the need for a commode (if the lavatory is upstairs).

Managing an end-of-life breathless patient at home: the ideal versus the reality

Most clinicians would like to help those who wish to die at home to achieve this but it is not a simple task. The national End of Life Care Strategy has set out ambitious aims for those caring for people at home and has codified these into a number of standards (End of Life Care Strategy 2008). A number of different interventions and approaches to help meet these ideal standards have been set out earlier in this chapter. However, when working with individuals and their families, it is likely that the reality will not always match the ideal. It is the job of the clinicians involved to devise a strategy that will meet the needs of individuals where they are, and in the situation in which they find themselves, rather than following an algorithm in a set order. This section offers some suggestions on how to implement the best possible care in less than ideal circumstances. For each aspect of care, the ideal is described, followed by the reality, suggested actions and the best possible outcome. The aim is to show how the gap between the ideal and the reality may be at least partially bridged.

Understanding the prognosis

Ideal

Both patient and family understand the prognosis – in other words, that the patient could die either suddenly or after a rapid decline or complication (e.g. due to an infection) and that this is likely to happen within the next year.

Reality

Patients with non-malignant disease often do not understand how serious their condition is. They probably feel that the illness is horrible or a nuisance but they may not believe it is life-threatening. This may be true even when they have been in hospital and had ‘near death experiences’ on a number of occasions. This can be true even when the clinicians caring for that patient think it is obvious that the patient is not very well and deteriorating. A patient and their family can remain unaware of how serious the condition is, even when death is expected within days by clinicians.

Suggested actions

- The first time you meet a patient, even if they are very well known to clinical services, gently explore their understanding of their diagnosis and prognosis.
- If the patient feels that they have an unpleasant symptom or condition, but have a normal life expectancy, begin the discussion about what can happen if things do not go so well for them.
- Help them to understand that they have a serious condition and it is important that they make plans for their treatment under different circumstances.
- Individual judgement will be needed to assess whether the patient is using 'helpful denial' or whether they really have no idea how serious the situation is, and when the latter is unhelpful for all concerned.
- If denial is an important part of their defence against overwhelming anxiety, you need to adjust your conversation accordingly.
- Useful denial can still be maintained even when making plans for deterioration and being cared for at home in the event of this.

Best outcome

The patient may or may not accept that they have a serious condition but at least you will be able to arrange to get extra practical support into the home and to help the family adjust and plan for what is likely to happen.

Timing of referral

Ideal

Patients are referred early to palliative care or breathlessness services, when their condition is serious but they may still have months or even years to live.

Reality

Patients are often referred when they are already seriously ill and housebound.

Suggested actions

- Arrange for services to come in early on, and focus on getting symptom control and carer support right.
- Increase contacts with services such as hospice community teams to get the maximum help in quickly.

Best outcome

Breathlessness services will make contact with the family as quickly as possible and, within 48 hours to a week, effective symptom control will be in place. The patient will be much more comfortable physically, with better control of breathlessness, and the family will feel much more supported.

Initiating end-of-life planning

Ideal

End-of-life planning is already under way. In other words, the patient knows where they want to die if possible, the type of support they would like to help them achieve that, and the sorts of treatment options they would accept (such as intravenous antibiotics) and those they would not (such as intermittent positive pressure ventilation).

Reality

Many clinicians and certainly the majority of patients will not rush to get involved in end-of-life planning. Some patients may feel it equates to 'expecting the worst' or giving up hope, and some clinicians will not feel able to broach the subject. It is clearly more difficult to prognosticate and decide when to broach the subject of end-of-life with patients who have non-malignant disease but it is essential. It is often best to use a 'hope for the best, plan for the worst' approach, as described earlier (see page 166).

Suggested actions

- Start talking about planning for when the patient is less well.
- Record how the patient would like their treatment to be conducted if/when they are less well as soon as possible after you meet the patient and family, particularly if they have indicated that they do not want to go back into hospital.
- A blunt discussion about end of life is not a humane approach, particularly

as a 'tickbox exercise', but broaching the difficult issue of being less well is something that patients expect clinicians to do at an appropriate time.

- Include end-of-life planning as part of the overall action plan or plan of management so it is seen as an integral part of care and one in which the patient is actively involved from the start.

Best outcome

The patient and their family will be reassured that services are in place that will allow the patient to have the sort of care they want when they are less well, whether it is at home, in hospital, in a nursing home or hospice, with respite care (where available), with palliative care services or with their medical team. They will also be reassured that adequate medication and other equipment will be available in the home so there is no concern at weekends about getting the support they need. The patient and family will know that everyone involved in their care is aware of what they want so they won't have to be 'assertive' at a difficult time or 'fight' to stay at home (when a less experienced and unfamiliar clinician feels they 'have' to admit them). The patient's end-of-life plans will be written down clearly in the notes and communicated to all caring agencies looking after that patient. In some parts of London there will be an electronic record (Co ordinate my Care) that will facilitate this. In other areas, there may be access to electronic medical records, but these are the exceptions. End-of-life planning will lead to the care that the patient wants as they deteriorate, and the plans will be modified as the disease progresses, according to the patient's wishes. All changes will be communicated to all agencies looking after that patient, including out-of-hours services.

Dealing with the family's feelings about end-of-life care

Ideal

The family will support the idea of the patient dying at home.

Reality

Many families are frightened of the idea of someone dying at home. Over the last 50 years, home death has become a very rare occurrence. People don't like the idea of a room or a bed being the one where someone they loved died. They worry about whether they will be able to use the room afterwards. This is very important from a cultural point of view. For example, some Chinese families will not want a relative to die at home, as they may feel it is unlucky. Do not make assumptions, even within one ethnic group, but be prepared to question the family privately about their attitudes to death at home.

Suggested actions

- You cannot, and should not, of course, force people to accept the idea of home death, however much it is now being promoted as 'the ideal' or simply because it is seen as desirable by the management of your commissioning organisation.
- If the patient and family want different things, you may be able to compromise. If not, you may be able to use services to relieve the family, while still helping the patient achieve what they want. Sometimes it is not a failure if the patient spends a lot of their last months/days/weeks at home but actually dies in a hospice or even a hospital, if they prefer that to dying at home.
- It is important that, as clinicians, we do not have fixed ideas about what patients and families should want.
- Work towards what the patient and family want, bearing in mind and being honest about what can be provided within the limits of local resources. Help patients and families plan to use other resources if necessary (either private or within the wider family) to achieve their goals.
- As the patient gains confidence in the team looking after them, they may change their mind about where they want to be cared for. This may also happen with family members, as some families may have felt badly let down and isolated in the past.

Best outcome

The patient and family will feel properly 'looked after and supported' at a time of huge emotional stress and worry, and there will be no unnecessary emergency admissions because of physical or emotional distress. A family that was previously lacking in confidence will feel able to manage their loved one dying at home because they have adequate services and support in place. Alternatively, the patient and family will accept their differences and the family will be prepared to accept extensive help from services to enable the patient to achieve their desire.

Summary

Patients who are breathless and who want to die at home are often prevented from doing so. Sadly, many are admitted to hospital as emergencies in the last days or even hours of life. It is likely (though not proved) that this could be avoided if there was early access to expert help, with symptom control for breathlessness, in those with advanced illness. The longer the time over which services have contact with the family, the more likely it is that emergency admission will be avoided, because there will be:

- **Adequate symptom control**: Breathlessness is frightening (both to experience and to observe) and clinical services are often unsure how to manage it. This can lead to out-of-hours emergency admissions.
- **Prevention of carer exhaustion**: The carers of those with breathlessness are often elderly. Even for the young and fit, taking on all the extra tasks that a breathless patient can no longer manage, watching them live (and then die) with a distressing symptom, and managing all other household tasks, can be utterly exhausting and demoralising.
- **Adequate equipment in the house**: The right equipment at the right time can make a huge difference to a patient's independence (raising morale and sparing the carer) and at the end of life it can enable someone to stay in their own house, if not their own bed.
- **Self-management strategies**: Learning some self-management strategies can help mitigate the impact of the symptom, reducing anxiety and leading to better morale, possibly reducing stress and enabling someone to stay at home.

Table 11.1:
Non-pharmacological interventions that can be used with a patient at home

Non-pharmacological technique	Benefits	Interventions	Best outcome	Limitations/ problems
Positioning	Encourages energy conservation by preventing bad posture Supports accessory muscles to help recover from breathlessness Facilitates more efficient working of diaphragm	Encouraging forward-lean position in sitting or standing Encouraging elevated side-lying position in bed Provision of powered or manual backrests on bed to allow optimum positioning at night	Patient has an effective strategy to aid recovery from/ ease breathlessness	Patients experiencing pain or extreme weight loss may have difficulty adopting a comfortable forward-lean or side-lying position
Breathing control	Encourages the patient to breathe more efficiently Aids relaxation and reduces anxiety Enables recovery from breathlessness	Recovery breathing technique Relaxed breathing technique Focusing on breathing out – counting breath out for longer than breath in	Patient has a technique to control breathing and aid recovery from/ease breathlessness Simple techniques that can be written down and used by patient and carer If utilised effectively, these techniques can reduce anxiety by controlling breathing and counter-acting the body's stress response	Focusing on breathing may actually heighten anxiety for those patients who are already extremely anxious – in this case it may be better to focus on relaxation techniques first
Energy conservation	Encourages effective use of limited energy reserves Encourages continued engagement in activities, in a different way	Simplifying personal care tasks by using aids (e.g. bath aids, perching stools, toilet seats) or altering techniques (e.g. using a towelling bathrobe rather than a towel for drying) Encouraging patients to learn their limits and stop before they become exhausted Delegating tasks to others Using a wheelchair outside when going out with friends or family	Enables patient to retain some level of independence despite decline in function Enables patient to continue engaging in some activities that they enjoy Enables the patient to be in control of what they choose to do and what they choose to ask others to do	Sometimes difficult to modify behaviour – 'if I can't do it the way I've always done it, I don't want to do it'. Patients/carers may not accept/ adjust to having equipment and may therefore decline it

Anxiety management	Gives a sense of control over feelings of anxiety and panic Gives carer strategies to manage panic or stressful situations	Explaining the body's response to stress and why the patient may be feeling certain sensations Identifying anxiety triggers and trying to address fears Having an action plan (written out and close to hand) to read through when breathless Distraction of thoughts Talking self through stressful situations ('I have been breathless before and I will recover from my breathlessness')	Patient and carer have a strategy to help control feelings of anxiety and panic Patient and carer have been given an opportunity to talk through their fears Providing knowledge reduces fear	Anxiety may escalate as the patient gets nearer to death Carer may feel anxious, which may exacerbate patient's breathlessness and anxiety
Relaxation	Helps reduce tension in accessory muscles used for breathing Reduces overall tension in mind and body	Progressive muscular relaxation Progressive neuromuscular relaxation Guided visualisation (using colour, visualising a scene, etc.) Encouraging relaxed positioning of shoulders and upper body Listening to a relaxing piece of music or visiting a relaxing place, e.g. a park or place they have enjoyed together	Can reduce muscle tension Can provide an opportunity for patient and/or carer to have protected time during the day as relaxation time planned and always observed Can be carried out in any setting	Not everyone responds to relaxation techniques May have little time to learn any techniques that work

References

Booth, S. (2009). End of life care for the breathless patient. *General Practice Update*. **2**, 40–44.

Booth, S., Silvester, S. & Todd, C. (2003). Breathlessness in cancer and chronic obstructive pulmonary disease: Using a qualitative approach to describe the experience of patients and carers. *Palliative and Supportive Care*. **1**, 337–44.

Booth, S., Moffat, C., Farquhar, M., Higginson, I.J. & Burkin, J. (2011). Developing a breathlessness intervention service for patients with palliative and supportive care needs, irrespective of diagnosis. *Journal of Palliative Care*. **27**, 28–36.

End of Life Care Strategy. (2008). http://www.endoflifecare.nhs.uk/support-advice/strategy.aspx

Spathis, A. & Booth, S. (2008). End of life care in chronic obstructive pulmonary disease: In search of a good death. *International Journal of COPD*. **3**, 11–29.

Spathis, A., Davis, H. & Booth, S. (2011). *Advanced Respiratory Disease: From Advanced Disease to Bereavement*. Oxford: Oxford University Press.

Appendix

Charities

British Heart Foundation
Greater London House
180 Hampstead Road
London NW1 7AW

Tel: 020 7554 0000

www.bhf.org.uk

British Lung Foundation
73–75 Goswell Road
London EC1V 7ER

Tel: 020 7688 5555

www.blf.org.uk

Marie Curie Cancer Care
Supporter Services Team
Marie Curie Cancer Care
89 Albert Embankment
London SE1 7TP

Freephone: 0800 716 146

www.mariecurie.org.uk

Pulmonary Hypertension Association UK
PHA UK
Unit 2, Concept Court
Manvers
Rotherham S63 5BD

Tel: 01709 761450

Fax: 01709 760265

Email: office@phassociation.uk.com

www.phassociation.uk.com

Professional organisations

American Thoracic Society
25 Broadway
18th Floor
New York NY 10004
USA

Voice: 212-315-8600

Fax: 212-315-6498

www.thoracic.org

British Thoracic Society
17 Doughty Street
London WC1N 2PL

Tel: 020 7831 8778

Fax: 020 7831 8766

Email: bts@brit-thoracic.org.uk

www.brit-thoracic.org.uk

European Respiratory Society
4, Avenue Ste-Luce
CH 1003 Lausanne
Switzerland

Telephone: + 41 21 213 01 01

Fax: + 41 21 213 01 00

www.ersnet.org

Global Initiative for COPD

www.goldcopd.org

Index